FLEX YOUR AGE

DEFY STEREOTYPES AND RECLAIM EMPOWERMENT

FLEX YOUR AGE

DEFY STEREOTYPES AND RECLAIM EMPOWERMENT

JOAN MACDONALD

with MICHELLE MACDONALD

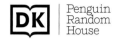

Publisher Mike Sanders
Editor Christopher Stolle
Art Director William Thomas
Senior Designer Jessica Lee
Photographer Sofía Fernández
Proofreaders Mira Park & Kristi Hein
Indexer Jessica McCurdy Crooks

First American Edition, 2022
Published in the United States by DK Publishing
6081 E. 82nd St., Suite 400, Indianapolis, IN 46250

Library of Congress Catalog Number: 2022934441
ISBN 978-0-7440-5924-3

DK books are available at special discounts when purchased in bulk for sales
promotions, premiums, fund-raising, or educational use. For details, contact:
SpecialSales@dk.com

Printed and bound in Canada

For the curious
www.dk.com

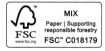

MIX
Paper | Supporting
responsible forestry
FSC™ C018179

This book was made with Forest
Stewardship Council ™ certified
paper – one small step in DK's
commitment to a sustainable future.
For more information go to
www.dk.com/our-green-pledge

CONTENTS

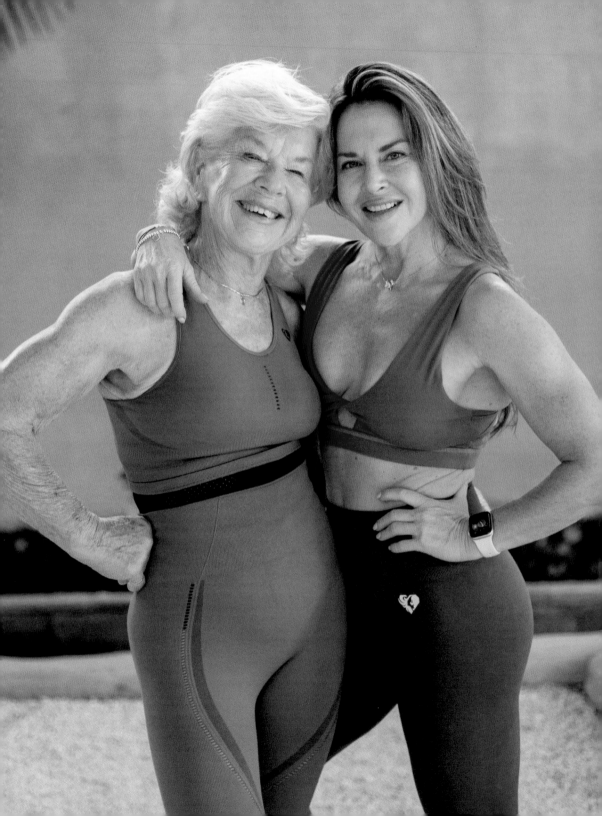

ABOUT THE AUTHORS

Joan MacDonald (@trainwithjoan) is a 75-year-old Instagram fitness influencer who's undergone a remarkable change in the last five years. She was on medication for high blood pressure and acid reflux; she had terrible edema in her ankles; her arthritis was extremely painful; and she had difficulty walking up and down stairs. Joan knew that if she continued on an unhealthy path that it might mean more health issues and more medications—and probably force her to move into a nursing home. But with the help of her daughter, Michelle, and The Wonder Women community, Joan was able to do much more than change her journey—she was able to help others on theirs.

Michelle MacDonald (@yourhealthyhedonista) has been coaching women since 2012, beginning with athletes getting ready for competition on the natural bodybuilding stage. She also started coaching women who wanted to have a major lifestyle change, working with them in what she terms "transformation groups." These groups became so successful that Michelle couldn't keep up with the demand and created a team of coaches for a program called The Wonder Women, which focuses on women's health and fitness. Michelle's most successful client is, of course, her mom, Joan.

ACKNOWLEDGMENTS

The publisher would like to thank **Jeannette de Beauvoir** for her assistance with helping Joan and Michelle write this book.

WHY FITNESS MATTERS

"

When you embark on a journey to transform your body, understand that the real journey is to transform your heart. Learn to fall in love with yourself and value the quality of your life, your health, and your thoughts.

We might start transforming from the outside, but the really amazing work is done on the inside.

You don't have to believe what you've been told. You can change the story. It's only true if you make it true. You have to rock the boat or you're never going to get anywhere.

Joan MacDonald

"

Joan MacDonald was an ordinary woman living her retirement years without much thought of bringing anything particularly new into her world when, during a visit from her daughter Michelle, she made a decision that changed her life's trajectory.

She decided to become healthy.

It helped that Joan's daughter is a fitness guru and chef known as Your Healthy Hedonista, who's coached women of all ages all over the world, helping them become healthier and stronger versions of themselves. Through her program, The Wonder Women, she offers physical transformations, allowing for a healthier, more vibrant, and more vital life. She took her knowledge from years of coaching athletes and brought that kind of program into everyone's grasp.

But it didn't happen automatically. What Michelle found—to her amazement—was that there was a significant gap between the coaching programs for female-physique athletes versus that of "lifestyle" clients—ordinary women who wanted to look and feel better for life. In other words, athletes and bodybuilders trained better, more efficiently, and more successfully than did regular people.

She set about closing that gap.

At The Wonder Women, coaches work with lifestyle clients in a very similar manner to how they work with athletes. All clients learn how to follow macro-based nutrition plans, improve their form in the gym, use progressive overload to achieve incredible results, and employ various cardio techniques to help drive their progress. The assumption is that a woman of any age—whether she's 18 or 80—is just as capable of mastering a few simple methodologies as an athlete. She can achieve incredible success by transforming her body and her mindset.

Michelle had been running the program for several years when on that particular visit she observed her mother's shortness of breath after climbing a flight of stairs and offered to take her on as a "client." Joan didn't agree immediately, but later that day, when Michelle came downstairs to go to the gym, her mother was waiting for her in the car. That was the beginning.

Years later, Joan is not only a fitness coach, but she's also an Instagram influencer who posts encouragement and positivity that can help transform millions of lives.

"In 30 years, I've lost myself, found myself, gained and shed countless pounds, and seen my three children grow up and create their own families," she says. "I've sold our family home. I've sadly seen friends pass. I've said goodbye to my beloved father and mother. I've had to learn more about myself and let go of more parts of myself than I could have thought possible. Now here I am in this last quarter of life, jumping into change with both feet and a much lighter, brighter heart.

"Who knew that at 70, I'd be embarking on such a whirlwind, joyful, tearful path as this? What I hope I can pass on to everyone is that even though we might start these sorts of transformation with the intent of losing some unwanted pounds and getting off medications, what we can end up accomplishing is so much more than that if we're only open to it. Truly, we can keep on growing, learning, and evolving no matter how far along the path of life we might be. I'm proud of myself and I'm determined to keep the torch lit and help others around me do the same!"

HOW TO CHANGE

Many people have dreams of achieving an amazing physique, lifting some serious weight, or participating in an athletic event. Those dreams are attainable—if you're willing to commit to making them come true. In a world where we tend to seek instant gratification and overnight success, it can be difficult to comprehend the amount of work that goes into achieving a personal record—or transforming your life altogether—so we shy away from doing it. But the rewards are myriad and long-lasting.

Are you one of those people? Do you have dreams of the person you could become? Do you want to change your life? If you do, Joan and Michelle are here to help.

Change doesn't happen by accident. It happens because you're dedicated to what you're doing. Dedication means effort. When you learn to focus on the task at hand and give it your all, then your success is nearly guaranteed—and you might even surpass what you thought you were capable of doing.

For those who rise to the challenge, a key factor in attaining a high level of achievement is routine goal-setting. Setting goals allows you to anchor yourself into a routine and into productive habits. Setting goals reminds you of how far you've come and where you're going. The result? Daily progression in the right direction that will eventually help you attain your dream: a life of health and vitality.

But before we get to goal-setting and dedication, we first have to consider why this all matters—to everyone. Because it does. Getting into an exercise routine does a great deal more than just help you lose weight. Physical activity can regulate your mental health, your sex life, your sleep schedule, and more. Staying active improves your quality of life and reduces your risk of developing a variety of significant health issues.

It also reduces your risk of getting sick. There's a whole range of diseases usually addressed through medication—medication that could be reduced or even eliminated through fitness: cardiovascular disease, type 2 diabetes, certain cancers, injuries, high blood pressure, high cholesterol. It's not accidental that the American Heart Association advises at least 150 minutes of moderate-intensity aerobic activity every week. Exercise does your heart good!

SAME WEIGHT– DIFFERENT BODY

"It's not difficult to understand," says Joan. "It's really a simple equation. It's about changing fat into muscle. I'm the same weight I was a couple years ago, but my body composition is completely different. You might think that 5 pounds is 5 pounds—but fat takes up more room than muscle. When you change that fat into muscle, you're essentially shrinking. So you don't want to think in terms of pounds. When I started, I was letting the scale rule me. A lot of people do. You have to find another way of seeing your progress. My scale says one thing, but when at the same time my clothes are fitting differently or I go down a size, that's what really counts. That's why it's important to do your body measurements and take photos and not rely on the scale as your only guide."

The key to the transformation Joan and many other women experience through The Wonder Women is simple: balanced, macro-based, frequent, well-spaced meals (and drinking a lot of water!) combined with aerobic activity and a substantial, sustained effort to build muscle mass through working with weights.

What this approach does, Michelle explains, is treat all bodies as athletes' bodies, with a focus on gaining muscle mass. What that does in turn is allow you to burn more calories—whether you're working out or resting—and gives your body shape and definition. (To be honest, that's what most of us are really looking for anyway—not just losing that jiggly fat but replacing it with smooth, beautiful, shapely muscle!) You'll look better, you'll feel better, and, ultimately, you'll live a stronger, more vital, and engaging life.

Athletes train against a performance metric that keeps them constantly checking their progress and challenging themselves to do more. "There's no reason why everyone shouldn't be doing that too," says Joan. "Taking your progress seriously is going to help you in the short term and in the long term."

It's true that regular physical activity offers immediate and long-term health benefits and improves the overall quality of your life—not just by reducing your risk of disease but also by improving your mental health. In study after study, exercise has been shown to reduce depression, anxiety, and mood changes. It improves focus, decision-making, and self-esteem. It increases muscle tone and bone health—both of which are critical as we age.

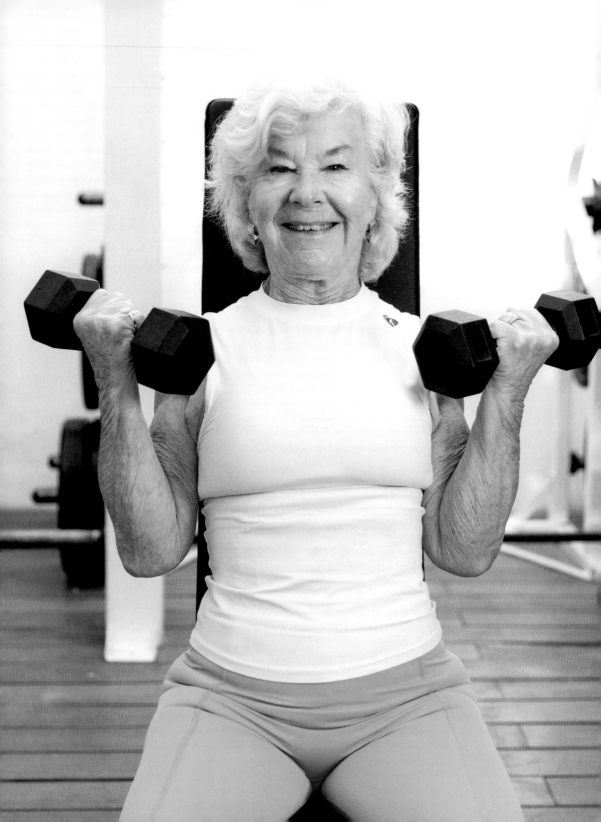

What happens as we get older is that we lose muscle mass as well as bone density and function. Exercise promotes your muscles' ability to absorb essential nutrients for growth and prevents muscle loss while preserving strength. It improves bone density and might help prevent osteoporosis and arthritis.

And, of course, as most people have experienced, being fit increases your energy levels and decreases your body weight—both of which work together to promote vitality. When you consider the benefits, becoming and staying fit seems like a no-brainer. There's an expression so many people voice: "I'm sick and tired of being sick and tired." If that's something you might say, then our stories and our insights are an invitation to you specifically, right now, today. Your past doesn't need to be your future.

How has fitness changed Joan's life? "It's in my way of thinking," she responds. "I'm more flexible. More creative. More open to suggestions. I don't take offense as easily as I used to. What I've learned has been so enlightening. Training does things I never thought of, things that can change a person."

And that new outlook does wonders for self-esteem. "It's reaffirmed all the time," says Joan. "Especially as women, we deflect compliments. I've done it all my life. I think I always suspected someone was making fun of me when they'd give me a compliment. My son-in-law was the one who said, 'Can you not just take it and say thank you?' He did that over and over again until I started really acknowledging that I'd earned the compliments."

That change has been one of the most difficult for her. "I still have trouble sometimes accepting compliments," she confesses. "I'm fighting a whole past lifetime of lower self-esteem. I remember one person telling me, 'You've changed my life'—and I didn't know how to respond. Are they just saying that? But I'm learning more every day. Now when people recognize me, I offer to have my picture taken with them! I can accept it better now, whereas in the past, it was very hard to do that. And that's because the better I've felt about my body and my life, the more I want to influence others."

Most adults in the high-tech (and mainly sedentary) world find themselves in the dark about how to eat and how much exercise they need. "If we'd been taught those things, we wouldn't have to be running to the gym six hours a day, five days a week!" says Joan. There's such a thing as working out too often or too hard, and that can be counterproductive. An NBC news report found that "overtraining occurs when a person partakes in too much physical training with too little rest and recovery after hard workouts. The resulting stress placed on the muscles, joints, and bones causes fatigue and soreness that ultimately affects performance."

So doing smart workouts is far healthier than doing too many workouts. And the right amount of exercise depends on a number of factors, including your age, your health, and your goals.

Still, as Joan and Michelle point out, all you have to do to get started is, well, start. "Walk a couple times a day," says Joan. "Do a series of bunny hops. Do three hour-long workouts a week. That's all you really need to maintain your health and be vigorous and happy." If everyone did that, she believes, we wouldn't be experiencing the obesity epidemic that's become the norm for many developed countries.

ASK AN EXPERT

There are so many myths out there about fitness and exercise and nutrition that we could write an entire book simply debunking them all. But one of the factors Joan and Michelle stress is this: The key to learning something new is to ask an expert. Your aunt Mary might have been a gymnast as a child, your next-door neighbor might have played football in college, but they don't know what your body, your situation, your present, your life needs right now. You need to find that out yourself and having the support of a trainer and a community of like-minded people is invaluable for making any transformation program you choose work for you.

"Fitness doesn't have to mean that you're an ultra-marathoner," says Joan, "or that you can perform 1 pull-up—or 100. Fitness can mean different things for different people. We need to look to people who know what they're doing, who've studied the body and know what it needs to be at its best. My daughter has been that to me. So has my son-in-law. They're tough but encouraging. That's the kind of expert you need in your life too. And the rewards exceeded even my most wildest expectations. Being fit—with everything that goes along with it—has opened a lot of doors."

She even accepts that she's now a fitness expert. "When my daughter gave me the Instagram thing, it was to get me out of my shell and keep my mind open and also learn from others. I never expected to be an influencer, to be famous. That's still a little hard to accept. But I can encourage more and more people. I can show others it can be done. I'm proof of it. We all need to develop differently. The key is to be the best version of yourself. This is the best you can be with what you've got. People with diseases and disabilities are trying. If you can be better than you were yesterday, that's great. Quads are competing in wheelchairs. They're fabulous."

MINDFULNESS

Creating a new life of health and fitness isn't just about your body. It involves being mindful about what you're doing. Finding flow in a world full of distractions isn't always easy, but this is one place where it really matters. You can incorporate that flow into your fitness routine to enhance what you're doing—and improve your life as a whole.

Mindfulness is about staying in the present, without judgment, to concentrate on what's happening here and now. "You can't focus just on the past or on the future," says Joan. "It's the here and now that matters." Most people have been exposed to mindfulness in meditation or even during yoga practice, but who does that as part of a fitness routine?

The first step is to have a purpose in mind. A long-term goal might be to lose weight, but that isn't going to happen in today's fitness workout or tomorrow's. Results don't show up overnight, no matter how impatient we might feel! So what can you do right now to stay motivated in this moment? That's your purpose for today, for this hour.

That purpose will vary for you over the course of time. Its specifics are less important than the simple fact of having a purpose and keeping it at the forefront of your mind. Your purpose might be just getting through the workout. Your purpose might be focusing on a given set of muscles. Your purpose might be a challenge you set for yourself for the hour. Your purpose—your intention—is what will allow you to not just complete today's workout but also look forward to the next one.

To be mindful in fitness is to pay attention to your body. Our bodies are always speaking to us, but we're usually too busy to listen or intentionally drowning out their voices because we don't want to hear what they have to say. So listen. Your body will tell you what it needs!

Being mindful in fitness also means slowing down. If you're throwing your workout in between an important meeting and a doctor's appointment, your mind is probably still back in the conference room or already forward in the waiting room. Don't let it go there. Slow down. Breathe deeply. You're here now and all is well.

Speaking of breathing, keep doing it. Intentionally. Breathing will help you deal with stress and keep you situated. If you find your mind wandering, bring it back to your breathing. That will always help you refocus.

"Mindset is a dominant part of this," says Joan. "Sometimes, you go through the motions and are on autopilot. Hours later, you'll wonder whether you did something. What happened between this and that time? That's not mindful. Ninety-nine percent of people aren't mindful, they do things automatically, they don't think about it. They miss so much in life. It's great when you know exactly what you're doing at what time, when you're experiencing everything there is to experience in this one specific moment.

"I enjoy more when I'm mindful. I know what it's like to go through life on autopilot. I've done it and I don't want to go there again."

Stepping off autopilot entails a willingness to communicate—and listen. "It's a two-way street between mind and body," says Joan. "You have to listen to your body—and your body has to hear what you're telling it."

Becoming fit doesn't remove the need to take care of yourself—you still have to look both ways when crossing the street!—but it will help you weather disease and injury better. "Growing up, I got everything. We'd pick up every germ and disease," says Joan, "and for me, it was always extreme. Mumps, chicken pox, and rheumatic fever twice that hit my legs and I had to relearn how to walk. It came on just like that—a snap of the fingers. I've lost my hearing several times and had tubes put in. I survived all that and it made me a stronger person.

"I fell—and honestly, I must have concrete for a head because I haven't split it open! I still fall, to tell the truth. I ride my bicycle around Mexico, and in our town, the sidewalks aren't straight. You can't take your eyes off the serpentine. I've had plenty of bicycle accidents here. It's embarrassing, but I just get right back on. It doesn't keep me from bicycling everywhere, that knowledge that I could fall again."

That willingness to literally get back up and keep going spills over into a number of areas. "There's a lot in life you could get nervous about," she says. "You've got to just not think about it. I don't put an idea in my head that this or that bad thing is going to happen because sure as shooting, it will! You can make problems manifest—and who wants to do that? My sister is always thinking of worst-case scenarios for everything. She's constantly worrying: What if? What if? What if? What you have to do is plan for the best, hope for the best, and roll with the punches when they come. Otherwise, you'll never do anything in your life. If I don't take a chance, I'll be stuck right exactly where I was before."

LIVING THE LIFE

Joan lives out her credo every day. For her 75th birthday, she went ziplining. She enjoyed it so much, she's already planning more daredevil activities for future birthdays. "People I know would be scared to death," she admits. "But it's fun, it's exhilarating, it's life! You don't need to borrow trouble. Just try to live."

She's still sometimes amazed at her own accomplishments—and popularity. "I hope my story can inspire others to get started," she says. "It's so easy as we get on in life to tell ourselves that our ship has sailed, that we're too old to learn new tricks, and that it's too difficult to make big changes. Don't believe a word of it! Big change—like what I'm going through—is a series of endless, daily triumphs over negativity and old habits. But the end result is growth, inner strength, and health. Every day, I have to get up and recommit myself to my new habits and my new attitude toward life. It's worth it. Saving my own life is worth it. So take care of yourself, learn to truly love yourself, and be the change you want to see in the world!"

CHAPTER ONE:

WHY WE'RE EXPERTS–
OUR STORIES

"

True fitness is about feeling healthy and being in sufficient shape to do the activities you want to do and live the lifestyle you want to live. If hiking the Inca Trail is on your bucket list, can you do it? Do you feel good after a day spent gardening? Are you able to climb all the necessary stairs in your life without getting winded or having to take a break?

Joan MacDonald

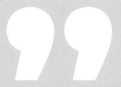

JOAN

There was a time not so very long ago when it took nearly all my breath just to walk up a flight of stairs. I still remember what that was like. I still remember how I felt when I couldn't do something because my body—the sheer mass of it, the weight of it—was getting in the way. It wasn't exactly yesterday, but it could have been. It was *my* yesterday. It might be your yesterday too.

My yesterday was filled with dieting—one diet after another after another. I put off doing things I wanted to do because my weight was in the way. I grew up in a household that didn't have a lot of extra money and meals were simple: You ate what was on your plate. What you saw was what you got.

At some level, I knew I was overweight, but I was definitely keeping my rose-tinted glasses firmly positioned on my nose. When I saw photographs of myself, I'd think, "It's just the camera." But there's no question that the weight—especially around my midsection—was getting in my way, interfering with my life. At any given time, I was lugging around an extra 70 pounds! My edema had gotten really bad. That was the first health consequence I really noticed, starting right after I had my last child—and he's now in his late 40s! I'd wake up being able to see my ankles, but by the time I was going to bed, my legs were really just swollen stumps, the edema was so bad.

I gained weight with every one of my three pregnancies. I loved being pregnant, I loved the sense of glowing with life, but I stayed big and then got bigger after each baby was born. And then I started thinking this was just who I was. That this was the weight I was supposed to carry. After all, it's easy to lose weight when you're young, but by the time I was in my 50s, I'd pretty much given up.

Fortunately for me, I have a daughter who never accepts those kinds of limitations. Thanks to Michelle, not only am I healthy, but I'm also happy.

I started out like many people, with a family that neither understood proper nutrition nor had a lot of money to invest in health. To keep things simple, we ate certain foods for dinner on certain nights. We had fish on Fridays (even though we weren't Catholic); other nights, it was meatloaf or baked beans. My mother baked all our bread—my father couldn't stand the smell of store-bought Wonder Bread—and I learned to make bread alongside her.

That wasn't unusual. Remember, I was growing up on the cusp of great changes in the world. When I was a girl, the small town where we lived was transitioning from horse-drawn carriages to trucks and automobiles; milk, bread, and even ice for the icebox—no freezers then!—were all delivered along the town's dirt roads by horse-drawn wagons. In the winter, we had to rush out as soon as the milk was delivered so the cream wouldn't freeze and push out the cardboard top. Sometimes, the breadman would forget to "anchor" his horse and then he'd turn away from our door and see his horse wandering away!

We bought our first electric stove when I was eight years old. I can't even describe how proud my mother was of that stove. I remember the time my brother chipped the enamel on it and she had an absolute fit. That stove was the first thing she'd ever owned that was new. She used a tub and washboard in lieu of a washing machine, and we made our own lye soap. It's easy to forget now how demanding daily life was back then.

I'm glad I have memories of how hard it could be, but I'm also aware that in many ways, it was fun, being conscious of transformation, of going from the old to the new. It made for an interesting childhood. Mom and Dad both worked because they had mouths to feed. No one in my family thought of going to university. My parents' main priority was to keep us clothed and fed—and what more can you ask for?

We were a large family and I was the oldest girl, which in those days meant that responsibility rested on me to look after the other kids. I was 16 when my last sibling was born, so I was like a second mom to my brothers and sisters. Looking back now, I was probably a little resentful. My friends were out having fun and I couldn't join them. Even though both my parents had jobs, it was still difficult sometimes to make ends meet.

Our house was so tiny, I honestly don't know how we managed! With nine of us at the table at dinnertime, if we were all seated—my father, naturally, at the head of the table—you couldn't even open the door! It was a house that was too small and a family that was too large. Junk food hadn't become widespread and we probably couldn't have afforded it anyway, but we did make ice cream from snow—that was fun! The cream in it came from my grandmother's cow. I did sneak candy from time to time when I had a little allowance or babysitting money—and I really looked forward to that candy. It was my "reward," or so I told myself, for all my hard work at home.

And we all know what happens when you start thinking about food in terms of a reward!

We didn't think then in terms of proper nutrition at all. We didn't think about balancing our meals. We ate what we could afford to eat and that was that. And actually, I *liked* a lot of what my parents did around meals. We ate very simple food and that focus was really ahead of its time. It's only recently that the world has rediscovered the joys and health benefits of simplicity. For too many people, everything is complicated, processed, filled with additives. Even not knowing what I know today, once I became an adult, I questioned how all those foods could be on the shelves and how they could be edible. It seems to me that preservatives play a big role in keeping people obese.

Of course, not that many people knew any better back then. I went to what was called "home economics" class, but we never learned about nutrients or balancing meals. It was all about how to follow a recipe. What good did that do? Who knew what was in that recipe? How could you tell what it did for—or to—you?

Even as a girl, even not knowing much about food, I always preferred quality over quantity. That's stood me in good stead since I've been focusing on my health these past few years.

We lived in Newfoundland then and a staple of our diet was wild game, which was plentiful: fish, elk, caribou, moose, even bear. People didn't think about any of this. They'd grown up eating what they could. Even though my mother was a waitress in Ontario before going back to Newfoundland to get married, she still didn't really understand about proteins and carbs and sugars. That sort of thing just wasn't on our radar. (Not that there was radar then either!) And, of course, like most other families, we always had dessert. My father called it a "stopper" for the meal.

Holidays entailed even more people at dinnertime for even larger meals. It was really important to us to do things together as a family and that's a tradition I've carried forward with me into my own adult life. Family is the most important thing in my world. There's tremendous diversity in families. You might prefer some of your family members to others, but at the end of the day, they're all yours. Did my family life set a pattern for me in later years? No doubt. I was the one who did all the cooking, all the cleaning, all the household chores.

But the truth is, while I was taking care of others, I was neglecting myself in the process. What I didn't know (and certainly didn't *do*) was the imperative to look after yourself first so you're then able to look after others. If you wear yourself out, you won't be good for anything. I remember so clearly that anything we'd now call self-care was regarded far and wide as selfishness. You should never put yourself first. You were there to care for your family.

This finally really came home to me when I was flying somewhere and the flight attendants came out to demonstrate the airplane's safety equipment. Should the oxygen masks drop, they said, secure your mask before you assist the child next to you. Wait, what? That goes against most people's instincts! It sounds so selfish! But in truth, it's the only way to save that child. You're no good to them if you pass out from hypoxia.

It's not easy to change your way of thinking. The airplane analogy stayed with me and I suffered when I saw the consequences my mother had to deal with. She'd always been one to make sure everyone else was taken care of before she'd even think of caring for herself, but that way of life takes a toll. When she got ill and eventually went into a nursing home, I was shocked to see how quickly she deteriorated. No one was helping her get out of bed to do any exercise, her meals were less than well balanced, and she had a lifetime behind her of telling people she didn't matter, so it was difficult for her as an older person to ask for what she needed.

If the notion of nutrition wasn't part of my life growing up, neither was the idea of exercise for exercise's sake (in other words, for health!). Exercise was built into our lives, into what we did every day.

My father's repertoire included a healthy dose of hunting and fishing. The men would camp out in the woods and they'd be gone for weeks, chopping trees, then tying the logs together and floating them down the river. I can only imagine the strength and energy that took! Exercise was built into his life as it was into ours.

Any other exercise we got happened through school. My oldest brother had the privilege of participating in sports, and he played baseball and hockey. But we all did something, especially in the wintertime when the pond froze over and we could skate or go tobogganing up in the hills. I did wish I could do some school sports, but there just wasn't time. I had to go straight home after school to take care of the kids, and even when we went out to do something, I had to bring them all with me. That got challenging!

So I don't know that my attitudes around food and exercise were ever very evolved—either through necessity or education.

By the time I graduated (we'd been in Ontario since I was around three), in my hometown, Cobourg, there wasn't a lot of opportunity in terms of work. The only people I knew who got jobs were the children of local professionals, people who had influence. I went looking, but I got caught up in the catch-22 of you need experience to get a job, but you need a job to get experience!

A friend had married and moved to Toronto, and she urged me to join her there, which I did. Within a couple days, I'd gotten a job as a clerk.

My supervisor, Mrs. Katz—I'll never forget her—helped me eventually get into government work. I was one of 3 out of 15 candidates who passed the entrance examination.

That's where I met my husband. I was in accounting and he was in the personnel department. I saw right away that this man could talk the legs off a horse. We used to talk for hours and hours. We got an offer on a house to rent in Toronto, although with the caveat that we were a married couple, so we got married. In 1974, we bought our first house in Cobourg (back to the town I grew up in), but that left him driving back and forth to Toronto for work. It was my job to get him up in the morning and out. And then he wasn't home until early evening. It was a difficult adjustment for me, but after Michelle was born, I secured a job again—this time as a clerk in the Ministry of Transportation. I stayed there until I retired.

My husband had a different experience from mine growing up. He had to become the "man of the house" when he was 15. His mother was a cleaner and she was often gone at suppertime, so there was no one for him to eat with. He wanted what I'd had. After spending time with my family, seeing us together at meals, he knew he wanted our new family to have that same experience. He didn't really know what a proper meal was. He'd been accustomed to putting spaghetti and french fries together!

And while I didn't have a lot of knowledge about food—I'd learned from my own mother, who was an instinctive rather than regimented cook—I loved to try out new recipes. My husband, though, would've been happy with the same dinner every night. For a long time, I did things pretty much the way my mom had. Over the years, I'd finally come to enjoy vegetables—I found my palate grew as I aged, became more sophisticated—but that still wasn't enough to keep me healthy. In fact, I'd faithfully copy my parents' custom of having different meals corresponding to the different days of the week. It might have been convenient, but it was a mistake. If you establish a habit like that, you don't have to think. Tuesday is meatloaf, so I don't have to figure anything out. In my own way, I was closed to change—and that's never a good place to be.

I had three pregnancies, and after each baby was born, I kept on a little of the weight. That adds up! In fact, it's no exaggeration for me to say that if I'd kept up the way I was going, I'd be in a nursing home by now. When you stop using parts of your body, they become atrophied—you lose strength and flexibility—and that was certainly how I'd describe myself at that point.

I did "try." I tried riding a bicycle. I looked down and thought the tires were flat. They weren't flat—it was my weight pressing them into the ground! I ignored it. I had friends who were more overweight than I was and I consoled myself with that comparison. I wasn't fat. I just needed to lose a few pounds.

What got me in the end was climbing stairs. They seemed to be presenting more and more of a problem. But that was the problem that proved to be my salvation: One day, when I was with Michelle, I tried to tackle a set of stairs and found myself huffing and puffing, and she immediately became concerned. And I'm so glad she caught me in time to change me and my way of thinking!

Of course, I had thoughts of giving up, but even from those first days, I knew I had to do it. I'm not a quitter. I'm just that stubborn. I've always

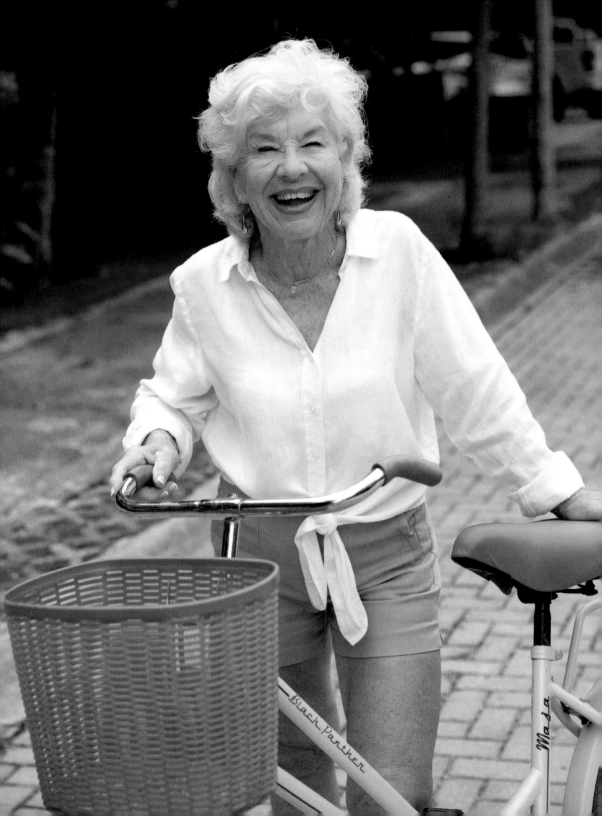

been stubborn, but it's a good kind of stubborn. I've survived things that might make other people want to curl up and roll over and die.

Stubbornness comes from commitment. When you make a commitment, especially to yourself, then you don't want to let the other person—or yourself—down. Someone is counting on you. And I carry that to the extreme, I think. I can't give up. What, it's hard, so it's not worth doing? The best things in life are hard. Deal with it.

Michelle is my rock. She opened my eyes to so many things. I have a daughter who has such vision and I wanted to follow her because she had the vision I wished I had. I believed in her then and I believe in her now. Michelle saw what I was doing and simply said "I can give you a better life." I'd been going to her bodybuilding shows, of course, and I saw what she was doing with other women. And a small voice inside me said, "If she can do it with strangers, maybe she can do it with me." I won't say I wasn't scared—of course I was! I was scared of everything. But when she said that to me, I felt this was it. This was my chance. This was a tremendous invitation into something new and scary and beautiful.

So when I was in Mexico at Michelle's house and she invited me to join the group, I found I couldn't say anything. I never really gave her a clear answer. She and JJ, my son-in-law, were going to the gym—later on, they built their own, but then they just used the local one—and I was already making excuses in my head not to go. Then I thought, "Let's see." JJ was already in the vehicle and I just got in and sat there, saying nothing. It shocked Michelle.

I remember finishing one exercise and then collapsing. I remember thinking, "I don't know what I'm doing, but I'll try it!" I know I surprised them with my agility in some of the exercises. As experts, they saw potential in me. It took me a few days to really commit. It was like learning a different language or being on a different planet.

When I returned to Canada, I struggled a little with the technology. Eventually, I learned how to print from a PDF and I learned how to watch exercise videos on my iPad. I was working out four days a week and that felt like so much time! And the weight—imagine it, back then, I was straining to get 20 pounds in the air and now I can do 40 in each arm. Who'd have thought?

I hope my story can inspire some of you to get started. You can create change in your body and in your mind. Change isn't one big event. It's a series of endless daily triumphs over negativity and old habits— and the end result is growth, inner strength, and health. Every day, I have to get up and recommit myself to my new habits and my new attitude toward life. It's worth it. Saving my own life has been worth it.

Even my husband has started training at home with weights and is starting to use the stationary bike and eat more meals with protein. You never know who you might positively influence! So take care of yourself, learn to truly love yourself, and be the change you want to see in the world.

MICHELLE

I always really loved my mom and wanted her attention. I didn't go through any of that silly adolescent stuff, thinking she was stupid or anything like that. Actually, I thought Mom was pretty great.

I was the only girl in the family, with one older brother and one younger brother, so I was always active in sports, even dancing when I was really young. I've always been something of an entertainer. I especially loved to make my mom laugh. But in retrospect, all the physical activity and having people watching me, paying attention to me, all that also started me on that journey of being in my body.

Dad was big on sports, but he didn't pay a lot of attention to my activities. I tried hard to excel so I could attract his attention. But my mom? She came to every single event, every single recital. She even had outfits made for them. And I did have a good childhood. I did well in school—and I loved disappearing into the world of books. I'm quite sure I learned more through reading books than I did in school or in real life. I read animal books, sagas. I guess what I really loved was being exposed to different ideas and concepts, reading about loyalty, nobility, friendship. I remember I'd be reading even as I walked down the street or up a flight of stairs. At night, I'd be under the covers with a flashlight, I was so loath to stop reading. I was the only kid I'd ever heard of who loved doing homework.

I asked Mom to show me how to cook. She claimed she wasn't very good at it, although I remember her making cookies, with us kids jostling around so we could lick extra icing off the utensils. But it wasn't just about sugar. We had a garden in the backyard and I remember picking lettuce, digging up carrots for dinner.

One thing I noticed about dinner: My brother got to watch TV with Dad after dinner, while I had to clear the table and wash the dishes because it was what the girls did. I rebelled against that notion. I was constantly asking why.

In fact, it's fair to say I was *always* questioning why things were the way they were. I was a budding feminist. I wore Birkenstocks in school before anyone else did. I was reading Gloria Steinem by the time I was 12. All that really set the stage for my life as a creative feminist.

I remember going on camping trips and Mom struggling with being overweight. It would be affecting the balance of the canoe or I'd be literally dragging her up the sides of mountains, but she was always such a good sport about it all, so supportive of the things I wanted to do. She was always willing to be there.

When I was in my teens, I developed bulimia, and even though it was clear she didn't understand what was going on, she was still supportive. The truth is, I was starving myself, getting dizzy at school, taking fiber pills all the time. I transferred to a private school for gifted kids, graduated early, and was at university by the time I was 17. Mom went to Toronto with me to see a specialist in eating disorders. I'm sure she had a hard time understanding me. I was pretty intense!

But not understanding didn't mean not loving. We've always had a good relationship and I've always been grateful for her. We're alike in that we're very independent. We weren't the kind of people who'd talk every night on the phone or anything like that. But supportive—that, yes, for sure.

A friend, a competitive figure skater, showed me about purging. The summer I was 16, I did it often. If I wanted to have a "perfect" day and then ate something, I'd make myself sick to get rid of it. That summer, I worked as a waitress at a boys camp, where there were a lot of social pressures. I was an introvert, intelligent, inquisitive—and there I was with all these 19-year-old counselors. There was some drinking and fooling around going on, and that just added to the sense of being in a pressure cooker.

Home wasn't any better. In fact, I was relieved when I was able to go off to private school. My family's dynamics were pretty difficult then. My older brother was a little out of control and had a terrible temper. He was a big guy and was always yelling about something. My parents were both exhausted. My dad dealt with it by being away all day at work and then going to the Legion Hall for a beer or two before coming home. Mom worked too, but she didn't have the escape of the Legion bar. She had to come home and clean and cook and do dishes and laundry. I was glad to get out of the house, but I was also lost and confused. I had to become my own adult very fast.

The eating disorder was disruptive to my life, but it taught me a lot too. It helps me in my current career because now I understand how people can be highly functional yet cripple themselves. You can waste a lot of energy trying to immolate yourself.

For me, breaking free was less about the food itself and more about becoming a resourceful, independent person who can face opportunities outside of her comfort zone. Instead of overcoming challenges, you discover it's too easy to go back to the drama. Things get so distorted for women. Living your life like that is like trying to drive with the handbrake on.

One thing that really helped me was yoga. I still believe it gives an incredible foundation for overall health and disease prevention. My path to yoga was more of a U-turn than a straight line. I've always been a fan of high-impact, heavy training, a real jock in school, and for six years, I trained and competed as a snowboarder in Big Air and half-pipe contests. I spent the off-season mountain biking and running, so by the time I was 29, my joints were pretty much shot and I had chronic acute tightness in my shoulders, neck, lower back, and legs.

Some friends dragged me to my first Bikram class and I ended up practicing almost every day for four months just to stay sane with my workload. I found I was getting so many health benefits, seemingly miraculous benefits, during those months that I started training to be able to teach. The experience was an eye-opener. I could see how, societally, women were more likely to have certain problems. All these women with issues around food and body image, they were checking their cellulite in the changing room. I couldn't hide from how disordered that was. I was a raging feminist who was observing women behaving as puppets because that's what their culture and their friends and all the TV and movies tell them to be.

It truly helped me break through. I did a breathing exercise, and during it, I saw myself through the veil of "not enough." I just saw myself, no judgment, just me. That was the beginning of my mindset change. That was the beginning of my journey into now. These days, I like a challenge, and if I fail, there's no attachment anymore. I'm like a kid, trying something, not mastering it, trying again, getting it right the next time. Figuring it out.

It's a journey that everyone is on. But I'd finally learned a way to cope.

And in fact, I really connected with the idea that true health is not just about eating more broccoli and exercising more but that people could benefit most from looking at various aspects of their life (financial, social, relationships, etc.) and integrating health goals from each aspect to build a lasting, solid foundation.

What I also realized was that my real passion with regard to nutrition was on the culinary side of things. So I started studying at the Natural Gourmet Institute, the only culinary school in the world based solely on whole foods cuisine, emphasizing the use of traditional, unrefined ingredients. I completed a three-month internship at one of Boston's best restaurants, No. 9 Park, working 13-hour shifts 5 days a week and really getting the techniques of speed, efficiency, and quality down.

During that internship, I decided to start training for my first bodybuilding competition and I've continued to win titles. It's taught me to look for strong muscle development, a certain athletic leanness, but to still focus on keeping a feminine and glamorous package. I won the prestigious USA championships in the 35+ category—at the age of 50!

I'm a feminist in the sense that I'm very conscious that being a girl has certain disadvantages. At school, the boys' sports programs got better practice times, more money, better uniforms, and, above all, better credentials. They were seen as *important*.

Even the ads I was exposed to bore out the propaganda: The guys all looked like athletes and the girls all looked pretty. I was very conscious of all that, all those ideas surrounding me, and it really bothered me.

Now, as an adult, it's my mission to see less neglect of women. Women represent a huge market, they spend money, and society has learned

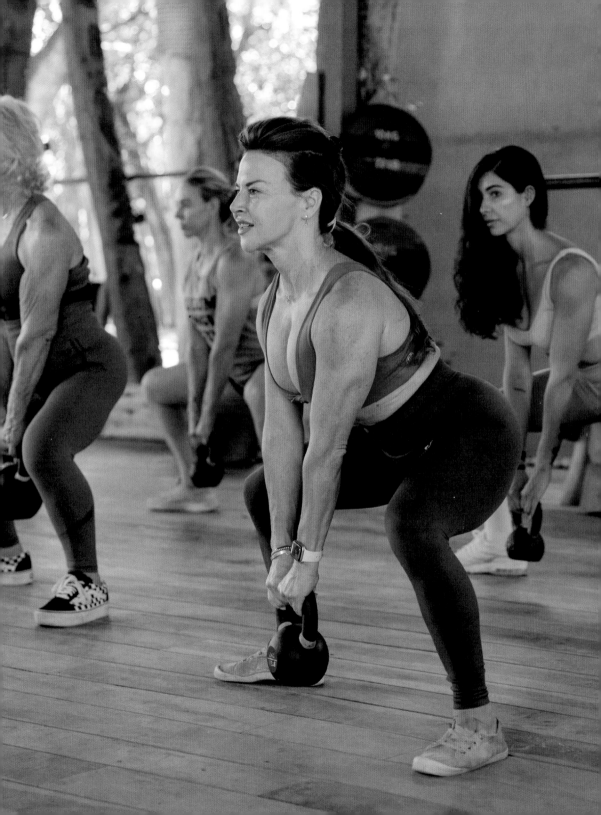

to capitalize on that, especially in terms of health care. Women have symptoms around their cycles, around menopause, and so their doctors prescribe medication, but the medication doesn't help with the underlying issues. Nothing has changed. Not really. People don't understand the female body.

So I set out to change all that. I was in the health and fitness industry, and I was seeing an overwhelming need not being met: the need women had for a coaching approach with science and experience backed by a focus on nutrition, training, and mindset. There was very little—almost nothing—out there for women who wanted to aim high and significantly impact their mindset, health, and body. So I created The Wonder Women coaching team to fulfill my deepest desire and mission: to teach other women my tried-and-true methodologies.

Collectively, we're creating a new narrative that breaks away from society's current story around women's health and fitness. Regardless of age, a woman can be incredibly knowledgeable and empowered around her health and self-care. We're allowed to aim high, build effective strategies to achieve those goals, and learn a process of self-awareness that allows for proper enjoyment of each part of a journey that never really ends.

At The Wonder Women, we teach the science of how to feed yourself, how to monitor your body, so you can have the energy and vitality you want. In other words, we teach women they don't have to be a victim of society's expectations, prejudices, and cruelties. They don't have to turn automatically to medication, which is in itself a culturally contrived phenomenon.

My own transformation started, as I mentioned, with yoga. I taught it. I practiced it competitively. My journey through yoga was intense and taught me what a powerful health modality it can be. Of course, at that level, there are some crazy postures. You're learning to control your body and your breathing at a very high level. I love yoga, but as I looked around the classes, I found myself wondering, "Is this all there is?" People in the room didn't necessarily look all that good. There were girls who were thin but who lacked tone in their glutes, who still had all these soft spots on their bodies. How can yoga teach us how to age with the most vitality when it's not helping us become strong?

I went to Boston to watch a friend compete in a bodybuilding show and I looked at these women, all of them beautiful, strong, radiant. They had tone and vitality, and I suddenly wanted that too—not just for myself but for any woman. What system provided this kind of result? I asked my friend about it and she referred me to her coach. I hired him (and, later on, married him—but that's another story!), and even early on in my program, I could see wonderful changes in my body.

My husband taught me about food—and remember, I was already a chef, but he opened up ways of balancing food that were so complementary to what I already knew that they were easy to practice. What started out as a portion control program evolved into the macros we use now. He wrote great programs and the results were clear: In only a few months, my legs popped—and that was on a 40-year-old! It obviously worked.

I started a blog: Your Healthy Hedonista. I love food, I was a chef, and now I wanted to marry the bodybuilding approach to food with eating well. And it all came together so naturally. It's so easy to get too uptight. If you know the rules of engagement, then you can allow yourself to draw outside the lines, to have some flexibility. What you need—all you need—is a way to chart your progress. Don't get caught paying interest. People see exercise and nutrition as a chore, and I'm proof positive that they're not. I love life. You can be fit *and* fit it all in!

As I continued writing my blog and including photographs of my progress, women started contacting me, asking me to coach them. I asked my husband to help me create the program and decided to get 10 people together. The group aspect of it was important from the start. We find that's the best way to keep everyone accountable and supported.

The hardest part is the mind. Once you conquer that, the rest will follow. You have to accept there are rules. You have to show up for meetings, you have to do assignments, you have to check in. Every week, participants took photographs of themselves and assembled them into an ongoing collage. It was a six-month commitment, and by the third month, everyone's collages were showing changes.

So the experiment worked! That became my transformation program, and it grew and grew from there. It works because it's a natural program. We do macros rather than meal plans. We take a slightly different approach to every aspect of fitness and well-being.

The odd thing was, people didn't want to leave when their programs ended. So we expanded. Past clients trained and became certified online coaches. Every year, we have to certify 10 new coaches to keep up with the demand. As of this writing, there are 1,500 people on the wait list and 3,000 people on the mailing list.

So now I had a business helping women transform their bodies, their minds, and their lives. And maybe that made it harder to see my mother struggling with all these same issues. But by the time I was in my 30s and early 40s, I'd started noticing that Mom was getting depressed. It was hard for her to even muster energy to chat with me. And I knew how serious that was.

Mom had been on diets ever since I could remember. As a kid, you don't pay too much attention to that kind of thing. You have your own issues, separate from the issues of the adults around you. I knew she had a scale and she'd been trying to lose weight. As I got older, I understood that weight was an issue for her, but I didn't have much clarity around that until it became a health risk.

So there was Mom, doing diets my whole life, and here I was, a chef and a bodybuilder and a fitness expert! My husband and I have to chuckle sometimes because she'll say she wasn't "that" big, but there are boxes and boxes of photo albums that proclaim otherwise. But that's not really surprising. I think it happens to a lot of women. Weight and lack of fitness creep slowly into your life, and most women who say they "suddenly" put on a lot of weight are generally not seeing their lives very clearly.

Menopause in particular is seen as a time for that kind of change. A lot of people have long-established bad habits, but when they were younger, there was a buffer to those habits. Unfortunately, that buffer fades with age and we see the effects of those bad habits compounded. What you were doing before menopause has long-term effects. And most people don't realize that because they don't turn to experts. They don't ask questions. They just stay on the same track they've always been on. They accept what comes to them.

When I'm traveling, I'm often the only one on the airplane to bring my own food—to make sure I'm eating properly. People just don't think about that kind of thing.

The proper way to be healthy and energetic is the one already practiced by bodybuilders: small meals, supplements, and train, train, train. That approach to life never really went mainstream—and it should. It's what allows you to lose fat and gain muscle—and do it naturally. No steroids—just a practice.

And this was the practice I was going to teach my mother.

I sat down with her for about two hours and we had a difficult conversation. I said: "I can help you. I'm one of the top transformation coaches in the world. But I need you to join this group."

I'd been feeling like I'd lost my mother—the mother I remembered. But I knew I could get her back and that she'd be even better than before. I knew I could help. I'd been coaching all these transformations and I knew it worked. I told her: "There's a line of people paying $3,000 to work with me, but I'm giving it to you for free. There's your added incentive." She was so deep in a pit that I knew she didn't believe anything could change. She just had no gas in the tank to think about starting a journey.

So I talked to her about God. "Your body is a gift from God. One of your tasks is to take care of that body. The before/after photos we do are inspiring. You can make your transformation an inspiration for others. We have to share what's possible with other women. If we're going to change the world, we have to shine a bright candle."

My husband was very invested in helping Mom, and eventually, I learned that working with her was the best gift I could have given myself—as a coach and as a daughter. My mother had never given up on me and I wasn't about to give up on her. We worked together on developing tools to help others who are struggling. She always wants to be thinking of others, of how to help them succeed.

What it's meant for me has underlined that I'm on a journey between coach and athlete, between coach and client. My mother is another client and it's been great to see this thing happening to her. The results don't lie. I see how hard she works in her training. That's an inspiration. It makes it wonderful to work with her. She's actually one of my best clients because she works so hard.

Speaking as a daughter, it's been an interesting role reversal with us. *You created me to be this person who can be here for you now.* A huge part of her ability to persevere is her mindset. She and my father don't talk deeply about things, but that's precisely what she needs, so it's what I need to do: Ask challenging questions and come up with new solutions to old problems. We have an ongoing conversation about who she is, why, and what she wants to change.

TRANSFORMATION

This isn't a story about a successful diet. It's not a story about losing weight and then going back to sitting on the sofa all day. To become healthy at any age—but particularly past menopause and on into the later years—it's a true life *transformation* that has to happen.

And the best part is, you'll feel *so good* living a transformed life!

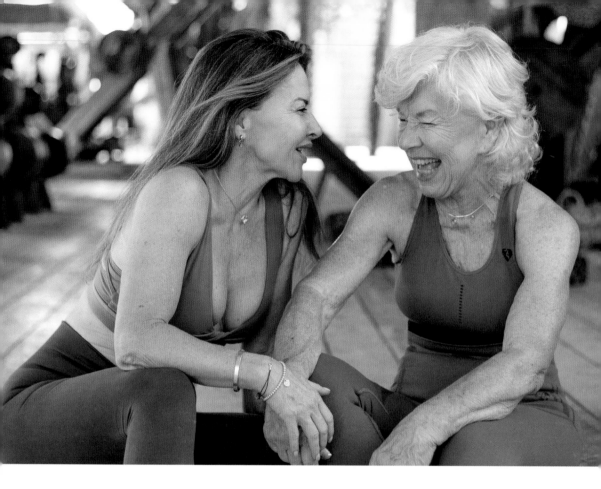

Michelle talks about this way of life as a "practice"—a term that's often associated with either a profession or a meditation. But the practice of staying healthy—eating right, exercising, remaining involved and curious about the world, finding a supportive community—is something within everybody's reach. Once you have a commitment to keep doing something, it becomes a practice. And the practice then becomes a way of life. And the way of life then becomes your identity.

"So whatever you need to be doing right now to achieve your dreams: Focus, give it your best shot, and reap the satisfaction of knowing you did everything you could to make it happen," says Joan. "This is the only life you've got. Make the most of it!"

Sarah Archie

I started following Michelle on social media years ago. I'd always been interested in weightlifting and healthy eating, and I'd even worked with a few trainers in the past. But then I started to have some health issues. I was eventually diagnosed with hypothyroidism, which affects so much of your body.

I struggled to get my weight off and had hit the big 40 in terms of my age. I felt my body had changed and what I'd done in the past just wasn't working for me anymore. And I didn't want to just accept that those changes had to happen!

I recall seeing Michelle's posts on her mom Joan, so I started following Joan too and watching *her* transformation was a huge "a-ha!" moment for me. I knew if Joan could transform her body in her 70s, then by golly, I could too. That's when I messaged Michelle on Instagram and eventually was accepted and enrolled in her six-month transformation program.

That was three years ago and I'm still going strong. Michelle teaches that we're really our own biggest obstacle and she focused a lot on mindset. The sky really is the limit, regardless of age, and she helps guide you through nutrition and lifting form. You begin to feel empowered and those shifts just transfer over to other aspects of your life and even to those around you!

I went on to win my first amateur bikini competition last summer. To be honest, that's something I might've thought was possible pre-kids and in my 20s. Michelle taught me to dream big. She teaches that age is just a number and that mostly I needed to get out of my own way! She was right, and these days, I use Joan's transformation all the time—for myself and as a way to inspire others. You can achieve anything you want to if you just stop telling yourself that you can't—and then just get to work!

I'm very grateful for all I've learned from those two amazing women. They're truly changing the world one woman at a time!

CHAPTER TWO:

MOTIVATION

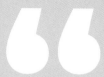

When people say 'You've changed my life. You've given me hope,' that makes me want to do better. When I think about stopping, that keeps me going. So many people would be lost if I didn't help them find the way.

Joan MacDonald

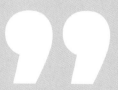

The most important factor in effecting transformation is your mindset. To succeed, you need to face your barrier stories, observe your negative patterns—and then disrupt them with a new internal narrative.

What's a barrier story? It's the story you've been telling yourself about yourself, the story that's forming a barrier between who you are and who you want to be. We all have a voice inside that warns us not to try something new: "I can't exercise because I'm too old." "I can't do a sustained program because I don't have time." "I can't ever become the person I wish I was." "My family would never put up with me putting myself first." "I'm not worth it."

The first thing to transform is that story. Try visualizing yourself a year from now. See yourself taking on new challenges, spending more time with other people, moving through your days with confidence and assurance. This is your story now. This is the life you know you've been aching for. And you can achieve it.

Everyone has a mixed past: some good choices and some not so good ones. We all have chapters in our story that aren't attractive, things we're not proud of, failures we've sustained. But that story doesn't need to be retold. It's over. You don't have to dwell on those chapters. You can let go of them. All you need is to give yourself permission.

In fact, you can always change the story because you're its principal author. No matter how old you are today, you have the whole rest of the book yet to write!

Your new story is the story of a way of life, not a temporary fix. It's deciding that you're worth it. That your family will deal with the changes.

That you're never too old or too out of shape or too time-pressed to attain a life of vitality and joy.

It's true that a lot of people start transformational programs that incorporate lifestyle changes and that not everyone sticks with these programs. That's why from the start you need to accept that this is a different way of life rather than a means to an end. You'll find that this life itself is incredibly rewarding. It's a life where you won't be on a diet but will eat foods you love (and a lot of them!). It's a life where you won't have to drag yourself to the gym but in which you seek out opportunities to keep your body in motion and you'll look forward to your workouts. It's a fundamental change in the way you live, work, interact, travel, love—everything.

The only way you'll be defeated is if you lose the sense of this being a change in how you live. Changing your thinking from "I'm on a diet" to "I'm living a healthy, vigorous life" changes everything. This isn't a fad. It's not a temporary measure you'll suffer through and then it's over. This is a change for the rest of your life. But it's a change you'll love and a lifestyle you'll love living!

So ask yourself this question: What keeps you going? That's what you need to find—the reason behind your choice to transform your life. What's important to you? What keeps you alive and intense and moving forward? That's your motivation. It's the drive to achieve your goals. It's influenced by a whole range of things: how much you want to change, what you'll gain, and your personal expectations.

But at its most basic? It's what will get you out of bed in the morning.

GOALS

Setting goals falls under the category of motivation. Keeping those goals in mind is what keeps you on track with your program. "I really had no clear goals in the past," admits Joan. "I was living a life that was really just an existence. I was just waiting for the end. Now I want to do so many things and I just don't know if I'll have enough time! If someone really wants to change, they have to change the way they think about themselves. It's a whole mindset. Knowing what you were doing wrong and changing it. Enjoying the process of the change. Being happier in your own skin, loving what you've done to the point where you keep on doing it."

"Keeping on doing it" is the key. Big, sustainable changes don't come from one-time events. They come from applied diligence, from making a little bit of progress all the time, bit by bit, day by day.

Joan and Michelle—and the hundreds of women they've trained—agree on how to set (and reach!) goals:

- **Set goals with your coach/trainer.** The first step is to find the right goal for *you*. Are you looking to change your physique? Lose weight? Enter a bodybuilding contest? Run a marathon? Talking with your coach is imperative. Based on their experience, they'll be able to help you focus on goals that are realistic and sustainable. Creating goals with your coach also keeps you accountable: There's someone who's watching your progress, cheering you on. It's hard to be successful at anything if we don't tell other people what our goals are so we don't let them slip.

- **Make a plan.** Now that you know what you want, you need to create a map to get there. Again, working with your coach, put together a detailed plan identifying the steps you need for reaching each goal. Your coach has a lot more experience with success than you do, so make sure they're the one guiding your strategy. Goals require short- *and* long-term plans. Once you have clarity on your goals, you can work together to create and incorporate the best strategy for reaching them.

- **Practice mindfulness.** Make sure you practice daily awareness of your goals through habits and visibility. Remind yourself of the what *and* the why of what you're doing. Create a daily checklist of habits that will move you forward, such as preplanning macros (protein, carbs, and fat), workouts at the gym, drinking three liters of water daily, expressing gratitude, and getting eight hours' sleep. Add photographs and quotes that inspire you. There's no rule against making it fun!

- **Track your progress.** This is the point of the before, during, and after photos Joan and Michelle urge you to take. Recording everything makes goal planning and achievement clearer, and it allows you to see the places where you have problems. Keep a weightlifting log, a journal that records your weight and measurements, a step tracker, and, of course, a record of your daily nutrition. It's easier to keep your goals in sight when you see yourself achieving them!

- **Ask for help.** Make sure your coach is giving you feedback on how you're doing and share any areas you're finding problematic with them. This is also a good time to bring in your community, the people who can support your progress and your goals.

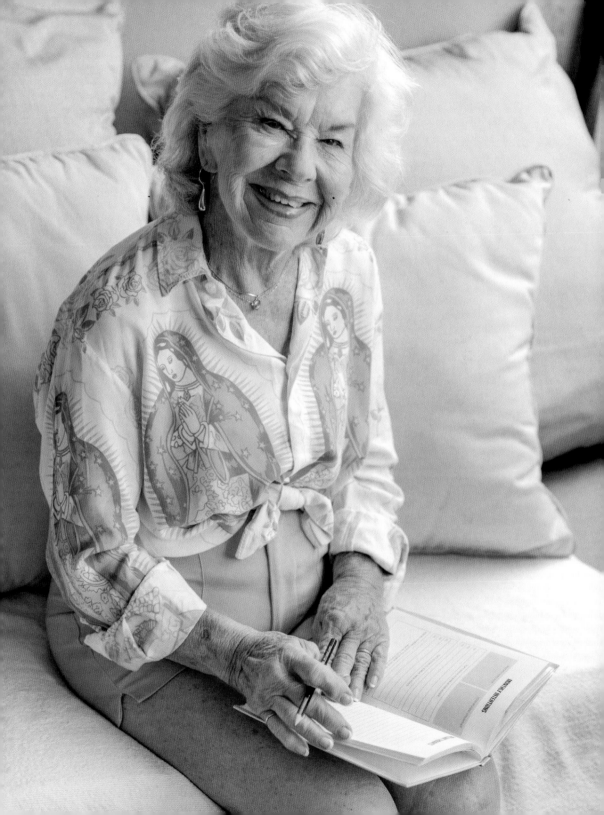

Joan says she never had thoughts of giving up. "Well, I'm not a quitter!" she says. "I knew I had to do it. I'm just that stubborn. I've always been stubborn and that trait has actually been good to me. I had all sorts of childhood diseases, and if I hadn't been that kind of person, I'd have curled up, rolled over, and died. When you've made a commitment to yourself, you don't want to let yourself down. I can't admit that I'm giving up. What, I can't do it because it's hard?"

That's part of the key to motivation: staying honest with yourself about what you're doing. Transformation isn't easy. Transformation doesn't happen overnight. In fact, it will often be difficult and frustrating. But you can do it. Not just in spite of it being hard—perhaps even thanks to it being hard!

"Sometimes, we get so fixated on where we want to be versus where we're not that our eagerness actually sabotages our progress," says Joan. "What do I mean by that? I mean that body transformation, especially a big transformation like mine, is going to be a very long, slow process. If I woke up every day expecting to see big changes, I'd be one very disappointed lady! I can't say it enough: Focus on doing the best you can with the day right in front of you and the future will take care of itself."

ATTITUDE

Your attitude affects your motivation and vice versa. The good news is you're in the driver's seat. You can change your attitude, develop a new, more positive attitude, and use that attitude to feed your motivation.

"We actually do the opposite of what we should be doing," Michelle says. "We're all systematically derailing our bodies' ability to be strong.

Humans are the only mammals that as they get older go through a decay that's completely a lifestyle choice. We think that age equates to frailty."

In addition to the problems inherent in believing that stereotype, older people might have decades of negativity behind them—negative habits, negative self-talk, negative perceptions. "They might even feel like they're old, so it's too late for them, there's not enough time left," says Joan. "But even if that were true, even if there are only a few years left for you, wouldn't you rather fill them with stuff that's interesting? Wouldn't you rather feel good about them and about yourself?"

And the advantage for older women is they have experience in weathering storms. "Bad things happen to everyone," says Joan. "If you reach my age, you're already a survivor. So turn those survival skills into something that can work for you!"

Monique Valcour, writing in the *Harvard Business Review*, cites "qualities such as persistence, being a self-starter, having a sense of accountability for and commitment to achieving results, and being willing to go the extra mile." That pretty much defines what we're talking about. It's through being positive that you can do this.

"Look at my photos," says Joan. "I'm smiling, I'm enjoying what I'm doing, I'm positive about the challenges as well as the changes. I know I'm not achieving my goals without having a positive attitude. Why even start if you're not going to believe in yourself, if you're going to think this is something you can't do?"

Attitude is a choice. You can always choose your response to things. You might not be able to change other people or the world, but you can choose how you respond to them. You can choose to take on your goals with a positive, cheerful attitude—or not. We don't have to tell you which choice is going to make success more likely! "If it's raining outside, you can get mad at the weather," says Joan. "Or, instead, you can bring an umbrella. You're not going to change the rain, but you don't have to get wet!"

Attitude also makes changes in your body and mind. A positive attitude will increase your confidence in what you can do. It engenders hope—and we can all use more of that! And as a bonus, a positive attitude makes you more energetic, more curious, more enthusiastic—about everything. You'll find yourself interested in doing more: traveling, going on an adventure, learning a new skill, meeting someone.

Like everything else in life, you won't always automatically have a positive attitude. No one gets up day after day feeling perfect. But repetition is your friend when it comes to your body and your mind. Keep reminding yourself to be positive, keep trying, and you'll find that as time goes on, it becomes your natural way of looking at the world and at yourself.

"Sometimes, it's hard for women to associate themselves with success," says Michelle. "When they start having negative thoughts, when they're self-sabotaging, I always encourage them to dig deeper into what internal dialogue they have going in their heads. You need to have a sense of urgency around changing."

Your attitude might not increase your motivation, but it will make achieving your goals a lot more fun.

THE MYTHS & THE TRUTH

For a lot of people, motivation precedes action. One day, you get up, look in the mirror, and decide that today's the day you do something about your weight problem. Or you puff up the stairs and don't like the feeling and decide you don't want to feel that way anymore. Or you have a health scare and it motivates you to get healthier.

Fear is a motivator, but it's not the best one because it doesn't last very long. A few days or weeks after your health scare, you might start to feel better and your motivation flags. Or perhaps the power of the mirror isn't always as strong as it was that first day and you decide the chocolate cake is just too good to resist or you don't really feel like working out today.

If we wait to feel motivated before we take any action, we might be waiting a long time.

Imagine you're sitting at home watching TV. We've all been there. And it's a real challenge to turn off the TV and get ready to go to the gym, isn't it? You're not feeling particularly motivated, so you might tell yourself you'll make up for it tomorrow rather than going today. But the odd thing is this: If you do turn off the TV and get up off the couch and go to the gym, you suddenly feel better. You're breathing better, you're standing up straighter, and—most importantly—you're feeling really good about yourself. That feeling is your motivation to go back to the gym the next time.

Motivation doesn't always precede action. In fact, more often than not, action precedes motivation.

What this means is simple: You just have to start. Just start and see how you feel, see what happens. You won't be motivated every single day. No one is. But when you're acting out what you believe, then things fall into place.

If you believe you have the right to be healthy and strong and vital and you spend your time on the sofa watching TV, there's a disconnect between your beliefs and your actions. That disconnect is uncomfortable and can eventually be destructive. But when you're acting in ways that support your beliefs, then your beliefs will become stronger—and so will you.

And when you feel tired or sad or weak and your brain starts saying things like "I can't do it" or "I'm not worth it," it's counterproductive to argue. The only thing you can do to counter negative thoughts is to take action. Go for a brisk walk. Do some sets at the gym. Remind yourself of your program.

Thoughts are surface things. They come and go. Attitude and action are real—and permanent if you commit to making them so.

Practices like visualization and habit-stacking will help. "Visualization is a great tool and what's even better is it can be done by anyone, at any time, in any place," says Joan.

Michelle agrees. "It can be a major player in manifesting the transformation you want," she says. "Be as detailed as possible in your mental imagery. Use all your senses. The more detail, the more real it will seem and the more of an emotional impact it can have. This is where the brain will develop a plan, find the open door, and execute. So often we think of just the body in transformation and achieving physical feats or goals, but we really know that it's the body following the mind's lead. Visualize to materialize!"

Habit-stacking is another powerful tool. "Pick habits that are already second nature to you, habits you don't have to think twice about, no matter how tired or distracted you might be," says Joan. "For example, if you always have a cup of decaf coffee after you have dinner and you want to start the habit of going for a 15-minute walk after dinner, then you can tell yourself that you can have the coffee during your walk. Again, visualize yourself getting the kettle ready. Wash your dishes while the kettle boils, then measure out your decaf coffee into a thermos mug. Get dressed appropriately for the weather you live in, grab your coffee, and away you go!"

MOTIVATION FOR TRANSFORMATION

The word that Joan and Michelle use constantly is "transformation." You aren't just losing weight or getting stronger. You're transforming your life.

And that's why it's so important to not confuse motivation with transformation. They can go together. But they don't always. If your training and nutrition rely solely on motivation, you're not looking at your life in terms of transformation. Because transformation requires the whole package: motivation, attitude, and action.

Knowing why you're engaging in this transformation can be key. If your reasons are important to you, then you're far more likely to be engaged and motivated. It's one of the reasons that before-and-after photos are critical to success: We tend to forget how bad we felt in the past once we're feeling better.

Specific motivation might change throughout our lifetimes—or even throughout a program. Where once you wanted better health, you might eventually want to go on to compete in fitness shows, try a new career, travel—the choices are endless. It might also change as you age. "One message I want to get out there is that us older gals can respond to proper training just like younger gals," says Joan. "Too often, people are afraid to push themselves, but I want to encourage you to start off with some simple movements, even supported movements, and work on your form and range of motions. Try to push a little harder and do a little better each time you train. Take some videos of yourself and keep a good training log. As you progress, you'll see your body changing, your vitality improving, and before you know it—you'll be doing the impossible!"

Action doesn't have to wait for motivation. It helps, but it isn't a prerequisite because if you act, the motivation will follow. "The good news is you don't have to believe in yourself to get started. The bad news is you don't have to believe in yourself to get started. So now that excuse is out the window!" says Michelle. "We can spend entire lives waiting to believe in ourselves, to feel ready. Thing is, belief doesn't happen in the waiting—it happens in the doing. Do that long enough and suddenly you'll find that the belief is there before the work. Because now you've set the precedent. Let go of the idea that you have to believe to do the work—and start embracing the idea that if you do the work, the belief will come."

DIET—OR LIFESTYLE?

"What it comes down to is this: Do you really want to change? If you're just thinking about an end goal, that's not about change. Anyone can lose some weight. But if you don't want to change your lifestyle, then you're just going through the motions," Michelle says.

Diets encourage an end goal: "I'll be satisfied when I've lost 10 pounds, 20 pounds, 40 pounds." When you reach the goal, you're done, and 9 times out of 10, you go back to the mindset and lack of action that you started with. The couch. The TV. The chocolate cake. Everyone thinks they'll be different—until they find they aren't.

"For me, if I want to stay on track, I have to change how I think and how I approach my life," Joan says. "It's an ongoing thing. It's living. I'm living the way I want to live, so I have to change the way I was acting before. Being more mindful about everything: what I eat, how I exercise, how I speak to others, how I treat the people in my life. It's all one package. It transforms your whole life. Why would you ever want to stop?"

COMMUNITY

There are tools you can use to help with motivation. "You can't do it alone," Joan explains. "You need someone to help and support you. If you have no one at your back, that's when you risk a big failure."

One of the women who participate in the The Wonder Women program writes: "I'm part of a Tribe of Women who support each other completely. We're worldwide and come from all walks of life. We stumble, we learn, we grow, we heal, and we continue to transform. We're living our best lives!"

One of the program's greatest assets is the community it creates with other women. Their backgrounds, their countries, their careers, their family situations are all different, but they come together in declaring themselves worth the work, worth the action, and in giving each other strength and support.

"We engage in behaviors consistent with our identity," says Michelle. "If you don't do the work to broaden the scope of your identity—more specifically, adopt, believe, and become your best self-coach—then your changes will be temporary. The real secret to long-term success is changing our identity and our beliefs about who we are. This will define how we live and what we do for the long haul. Just one simple way to aid that athlete identity shift is to surround yourself with others doing what you want to do or who are where you want to be. Watch how they move, how they stand, how they talk. Pick up on their passion for learning, for growth, for self-care and compassion, for a higher standard."

Creating a support system is what will keep you engaged and curious about the process. Just as Michelle advocates finding experts, you might consider finding a mentor, someone experienced in the habits you want to acquire. Having a coach, a trainer, or a workout partner will keep you going, even on the days when your own motivation is low.

And then, surround yourself with positive people. Positive friends and family enhance your positive self-talk, which also—bonus!—helps you manage symptoms of depression and anxiety.

That positive community gives back again and again. "We did a retreat recently, all the girls were here, and it was such a beautiful feeling," says Joan. "We need each other. They all got along, even though they all have different lives, different levels of education, but there wasn't a bit of drama. Men have that camaraderie; women usually don't, but this proved it could be done. The love that week was life-changing for a lot of them."

Michelle agrees. "People tell themselves stories about why they can't do something," she says. "That's normal. We all experience self-doubt. But being part of a group allows you to tap into a group dynamic so you're not in it alone. There's always someone there to help you get over any bumps you might be experiencing. Years later, a lot of the women I've worked with are still friends, still supporting each other, still helping each other avoid pitfalls."

Finding and giving that support is critical. And it might not come from the direction you anticipate. Joan found her husband wasn't the cheerleader she'd hoped he'd be. He even occasionally joked about her weighing food or insisting on her gym time. She didn't dwell on it. She understood we can only change ourselves—we can't change anybody else. So she relies on Michelle and on her many Instagram fans to keep her motivation level high.

"I see such good relationships in this group. They've got each other's backs. That kind of support is usually lacking in other relationships I see," she admits. "It's so much nicer to be surrounded by people who are really connected. It's such a different feeling. That's why I love being in Mexico with my daughter and her husband because they completely accept each other—and they accept me."

Becoming an Instagram influencer has widened Joan's reach and her sense of community. "When my daughter gave me the Instagram account, it was to get me out of my shell and to keep my mind open and learn from others," she says. "I never expected to be an influencer, to be famous. That's still a little hard to accept! But I love being able to encourage more and more people. We all need to develop differently. I want to encourage everybody to be the best version of themselves."

The community she's created with Train with Joan is deliberately positive. "You might not be able to do what other people are doing," she says, "but you can always be a little better today than you were yesterday. There are people out there with diseases and disabilities, and they're trying. They're doing their best. You might not be able to skip, but you can walk. You might not be able to walk, but you can do upper-body strength. Terry Fox was my greatest hero. He knew he wasn't going to last, but he wanted to impact as many lives as he could before he died."

The examples of para-athletes like Fox (who ran across Canada to raise money for cancer research) and others inspire Joan to be inspiring herself. "I really like the saying 'Pass it on,'" she says. "It really does mean something."

MINDFULNESS

As we've seen, the best motivation is anchored in mindfulness, which we talked about briefly in the introduction. Keeping the focus on this moment will help you stay away from guilt over the past or anticipation of the future. It might be more pleasant to dwell in the past or the future, but that's because you don't have any responsibility, any agency. You can't change the past and the future is truly the great unknown. So reminiscing and wishing are easy places to stay. The present is what demands responsibility. You can act—but only in the present. You can choose—but only in the present. So being mindful of every moment is seizing your ability to steer your life rather than letting it bob about on the currents of everyone else's actions while you dream of the past or the future.

Motivation often suffers when people feel they've failed or haven't done their best or are somehow unsuccessful and they forget to live in the present. Joan has an answer for that. "I'm going to try," she says. "You have to try. It's about not giving up. It's about persevering. I'm not doing it perfectly. I certainly wasn't doing macros perfectly for my first two years! But that didn't stop me. Now I'm doing the best I can and seeing success. I advise people to do it as precisely as possible. You can still make it work as long as you're staying within the parameters."

And motivation is spurred by success, even in the smallest things, such as how to prepare for exercise. "When I go in, I always do a warmup so I don't injure myself with cold body parts," says Joan. "I bike to the gym. Afterward, it's cooldowns and then job well done. I've accomplished what I came for. Even if I didn't want to go in, I feel better for doing it."

Keeping your goals in mind, even reciting them every morning or writing them on a notepad to keep on your desk, can be helpful. "Motivation is so personal. It comes down to this: What do you really want to change?" says Joan. "If you're just thinking about an end goal, that's not about change. 'Lose x number of pounds' isn't a great goal. If you don't want to change your lifestyle, then losing weight is just a motion you're going through. I know—I did it. And I know the difference. For me, if I want to stay on track, I have to change how I think and how I approach my life. It's an ongoing thing. It's living. I'm living the way I want to live, so I have to change the way I was acting before. Being more mindful."

Mindfulness comes into play when you first consider making a change in your life. What are you doing now that's making you uncomfortable? Can you sit with it, examine it, analyze it? Are you aware of what it's taking away from your living the life you want? "A lot of us are aimless, so you've got to do a lot of change within if you want to have a big change in your life," says Joan. "Be serious about it. Not to the point of not being fun but serious about incorporating change into your life. If you want your health, you have to work for it. You can't buy it—or get it back if you lose it. Anything worthwhile, you have to work for. It doesn't just drop in your lap. I still have to put in the effort. I'm lucky I have my community around, my daughter and son-in-law, but the truth is, they can't do it for me. I don't automatically get good health."

There's a strong connection between mindfulness and perseverance. "The problem is, people don't even think of what they're doing. Right now. In this moment," says Joan. "And that influences everything else. I just don't give up that easy. I wouldn't have much respect for anyone who gave up that easy. There have sure been moments when I wanted to throw the towel in, but saying it and doing it are two different things. There's so much I'd like to run away from—I think that's probably true for everyone. You have to do what you have to do.

"I didn't think my daughter and son-in-law really believed I could do it. I had no technical upbringing. I wasn't familiar with the tools I had to use. I know in my heart they didn't think I'd stick with it all these years. But they were willing to put in the effort to keep me going by whatever means they could."

And that inspired her to keep putting in the effort, to try things that once upon a time made her feel uncomfortable. "Investing in your mental and emotional health as well as your physical health is worth its weight in gold. Now I make journaling—as well as meditation and deep breathing—a regular part of my daily routine. It really helps spark my journey into more self-awareness and mindfulness, and it helps me structure my day so I make sure to create space for all the important things."

Keeping track of progress is part of a holistic approach to transformation. "You've got to do your best," Joan says. "What I was doing before? It wasn't living. I was just existing. There was a lot of crying inside. I didn't like my life. I had to see change. I had to do it for me, for my peace of mind. And now, knowing I can get through and make a change like I have, my friends can see the change. I also had to show them I could change."

KEEPING AT IT

Temptation is often the enemy of motivation. There are too many reasons around us as well as reasons we give ourselves to give up. "There's always that temptation to go back," Joan says. "A smell memory of a food can be really enticing, but when you know it's not any good for you, you have to leave it alone. And I can do that. I can say no to it for one simple reason: I don't want any part of how I was. I just want to live a healthy life, enjoy what I can.

"I still find technical stuff difficult. I'm not good at taking pictures. I need to take more of an active part in producing photos and stories and whatnot for the audience. Michelle and I might be on the same page in terms of the flow, but she's most definitely the brains behind it. I can see where she's going, but I don't have the insight to put it together, to see what she sees. But I know where I want it to go. When people say 'You've changed my life. You've given me hope,' that makes me want

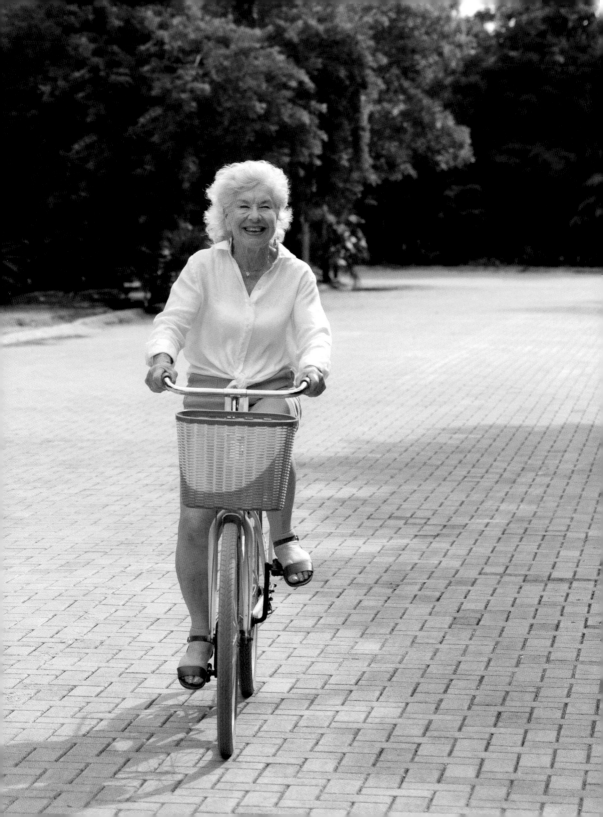

to do better. When I think about stopping, I remind myself that so many people would be lost if I didn't help them find the way. That's great motivation!"

Going back to the source, going back to your goals, is an exercise in motivation and mindfulness, and it can guide you every step of the way. "Ask yourself what your intention was to begin with, what your hopes are, and once you do, you realize that anything that's going to change is going to take time," Joan says. "You can spend your time doing nothing or you can spend that time doing something for yourself, even if you don't want to go through the whole process. Be honest: Do you really want to make a better life for yourself and can you take all the criticisms that will go with it? Because you can—you just have to believe.

"There's always a low point every month, a point of discouragement. I often wonder if it's hormonal. There might be a couple hours or a day I don't feel like doing it anymore. Those days, I just get on. I don't let it take root—and you can't either. Because you're creating something new and beautiful inside yourself. Nothing can stand in the way. There are black times throughout everybody's life when you can't see the light at the end of the tunnel. It's not a nice feeling."

Acknowledging your discouragement, your disappointments, your fatigue—Joan is right: None of those are nice feelings. But mindfulness teaches us to observe them. To take note: *Ah, yes, there's that feeling again. I recognize it. I've done battle with it before. I know it will pass.*

WAYS TO KEEP ON TRACK

Joan has suggestions for keeping your focus in the right place:

- Write down your routine by using a journal or an app.

- Change things around! Instead of saying "I can't," say "I'll try."

- Mindfulness helps keep you relaxed and focused.

- Don't do it alone! Find an expert to guide you.

- Review your goals. Seeing progress is a great motivator.

- Set new goals. Where do you want to be this time next month? How about this time next year? Work on a strategy to get there.

- Keep up the momentum. After three months, you'll have developed a new habit that can stay with you for a lifetime.

As we'll see, setbacks are normal, but developing resilience can help you carry on and pick up where you left off even when something goes wrong. "When you really start taking care of yourself, body *and* mind, you develop a much stronger relationship with yourself," says Joan. "You learn to truly love yourself unconditionally but also to start doing more of the things that bring you more health and strength and joy. And as a result, you crowd out the shaming thoughts, replacing them with loving thoughts. It's an entirely different journey. I hope you'll become the mistress of your thoughts and emotions and start living the life you always wanted for yourself. Let go of your inner shame. Let go of your inner critic. This time is for you!"

Terra Bautista

I'd reached a point in my life where I was tired. I was tired of pretending I didn't have an issue with my weight and I was tired of pretending I was happy with the way I had allowed my weight gain to spiral out of control, impacting and limiting me in many aspects of my life. I was avoiding social gatherings, photos, shopping—anything that would remind me of how much my body had changed over the past 20 years. I wanted to be around for my children and feared that my health would soon be impacted by my sedentary lifestyle and bad relationship with food.

I went to God and asked him for help and, in faith, anticipated he'd provide the way. Then I saw Joan and I was immediately intrigued by her journey and amazed by her transformation. Little did I know that her story would ignite a flame in me and lead me to where I am today! Thus, I began my fitness journey with The Wonder Women. My goal was to lose 40 pounds, but ultimately, I lost 91 pounds in 6 months, transforming my body in ways I never imagined.

It took laying all my excuses aside and accepting where I was envisioning a new me. It took getting out of my comfort zone, waking up at 4:00 in the morning to get my workouts in for the day. It took learning to love myself, choosing my health over food. People are often impressed with the physical changes despite the tremendous work that goes into changing the way you think.

I'm so thankful for the love and support I received from my husband, my children, and my friends and family—not to mention the support of Michelle and my coach Anni and the remarkable program designed to take women like me from start to finish.

It was a time of loss, healing, discovery, empowerment, newfound friendships, sweat, and hard work. I only hope my journey will capture the hearts of many, as did Joan's, and ignite hope where there is none.

CHAPTER THREE:

MAKING ROOM
FOR CHANGE

If you're looking for a change, I can tell you it's not an easy journey, but it is well worth it. I hope my story gives you the confidence that you can change too. If I can do it, you can do it!

Joan MacDonald

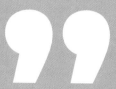

Change begins with one thing: a decision. You might not have even articulated to yourself exactly what the change is you're looking for. You might only know intuitively that something isn't right or that there's something bigger and better out there. But in the end, you must make a decision. After that, it's just about following through—and that's where this book comes in.

You can't just want to change. You have to decide to change.

Here are some of the thoughts that might be pushing you toward making your decision:

- I'm tired all the time.

- I wish I liked my reflection in the mirror.

- Will I always be around for my family?

- I want to have more energy.

- Is medication really the only answer?

- Something has to change. I can't live like this.

- I want to _____.

Now take those questions and ask yourself: Am I willing to make a decision to change?

Wanting something is fine, but it's often time-stamped: Your wants might change, circumstances might stand in the way, other things might end up taking priority.

On the other hand, making a decision involves action: It's about commitment and achieving forward momentum.

Sometimes, you reach the point where not changing is a decision itself. Not changing can be far more painful than changing, no matter how frightened you might be of moving forward. It's accepting that like it or not, this is the way things are. It's committing to being forever restless, forever frustrated, forever wanting.

And that's not healthy for anybody.

This is your life. There are many things about it that are completely outside of your control. You might have health issues. You might have had a difficult childhood. So much of what we experience depends on factors over which we don't have agency. But there are many, many spaces in your life where you can claim—or reclaim—control. All you have to do is decide.

So take a moment now and think about how much you want to change—and then make the decision to act. To do something about it. Whatever your reasons, once you've committed, you'll see your path forward more clearly.

What we're talking about here isn't easy. In fact, it's really difficult. "Michelle doesn't sugarcoat. She doesn't say it will be easy—in fact, she says it's really hard," says one of the program participants. "She doesn't dumb anything down. She respects women and expects them to be self-motivated and figure things out. And that inspires confidence."

Michelle wryly agrees. "Sometimes, I have to say hard things to people to get them to show up for themselves," she says.

It's a truism that the more challenging something is, the more it's worth doing. Another way of looking at it is seeing the challenges as underlining your achievements. Deciding to change your life is already an achievement and it probably came at no small cost. Getting up every day and recommitting yourself to that choice is a challenge—and an achievement. Every milestone you'll record is a challenge and an achievement.

Because, as an old advertising campaign assured consumers, you're worth it.

BREAKING FREE FROM WHAT'S HOLDING YOU BACK

For a lot of us, what's holding us back includes a lifetime of experiences that were less than optimal. The truth is, everyone's been on a diet—and everyone's failed. Over time, these diets have changed, as nutrition experts learned more about what's healthy and what can be detrimental in the long run. No matter which diet plan you choose, there comes a time when it just doesn't work anymore. You drop weight and then at some point, you regain it—often gaining even more than you lost! Failure becomes your constant companion and you start to wonder if you'll ever feel good about your body and your health again.

This is why in Michelle and Joan's program, the before-and-after pictures are critical. Most people discredit their own ability to have the results that the photographs make clear. It doesn't matter where you start. But when others see the "before" photographs, it's something they can identify with and relate to. And knowing that one person was able to move from point A to point B is a powerful indicator of how a transformation and cultivation program can work.

"Beyond transformation is the idea of cultivation," says Michelle. "It's the idea of imbuing your process with as much joy and as many personal touches as you can. We're taking your body and lifestyle mindset from a raw state and then you're doing the really exciting work of cultivating it."

I looked at Joan and thought, "If she can do it, I can do it."

Lesley Christensen, The Wonder Women participant

How does that work? "Say you just bought a house," says Michelle, "and it's not the way you want it to be, but it's what you have to work with. You're going to spend the first six months really just stripping it down to its bare bones so you can create the kind of space you want it to be. Once you've done that, you're left with a bare house, an empty yard. Now you can start building and cultivating what you want your home to look like. You take pride in the rebuilding, in deciding where you want the cupboards to be, what the décor will look like, what seeds you're planting in the garden."

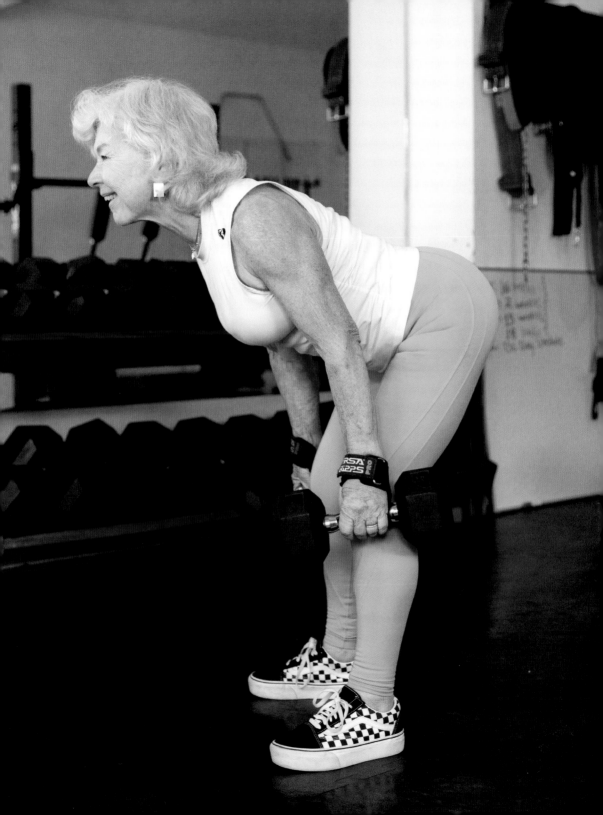

So think of your preparation just as you would preparing a house to live in—which is, essentially, your body. Where will you want to place emphasis? What will make you smile when you look in the mirror?

"Losing the weight is the equivalent of that first step of stripping everything down," Michelle says. "It's the dirty, hard work you have to do to create the tabula rasa that will enable you to do something wonderful, to find your style and how you want to move forward through life."

Joan agrees. "This was about finding my style," she says. "I have my books, my programs, my app, even the plastic surgery I had done on my eyelids. It's all meant I could re-create myself. It's enabled me to cultivate myself as an adult."

"The life you've created when you're 50 is the result of decisions you made at 19 or 25," says Michelle. Now you can have what she calls a breakthrough moment. "To have that breakthrough moment in middle age—that moment where you decide who you are—and want to start chipping away at that, it's just choice. We've been making choices all our lives, whether or not we're aware of them. Now is the time to ask yourself, 'Can I have a different choice?'"

These aren't necessarily big, sweeping choices. They're small, simple, everyday moments where you can be thoughtful about what you're doing. Someone coming home from a stressful day at work might habitually turn to the refrigerator or a glass of wine, but there are other ways of de-stressing, like taking deep breaths or doing a backbend to open your spine. There are choices that keep you in one place and choices that help you move forward.

"You can make that reflect the woman you've been attracted to—that woman who could be you," says Michelle. "Everyone has those choices. It's up to you to choose Door A or Door B."

And while these choices can be made at any age, people often think they're easier to make when we're young. That's not necessarily the case: Having lived through myriad other choices—some good; some not so good—women in middle age are often open to making a "now or never" decision. "Isn't it exciting to finally know how to slow down the aging process?" asks Joan. "Maybe what they need to be teaching us in school is how to take better care of our health. Eating more protein, avoiding excessive weight gain, and using weight training to maintain our health—all that could be implemented by everyone."

"Anyone can do it," agrees Michelle. "Menopause isn't what you think it is. We're told that women lose their vitality after menopause, and that's absolutely not true. I see lots of women in their 50s and 60s bench-pressing, deadlifting, doing all the hard things. They're really killing it. There was a 48-year-old woman who was working out once at her daughter's gym and the local football coach went up to her and told her she had a great technique. Age loses its meaning when you're healthy and doing what you need to do to stay that way."

Our culture tells us that vitality belongs to the young. "There's this social media story about menopause that drives me nuts," says Michelle. "They're trying to be helpful, but the medical narrative isn't the only one. You're no different. You're just going through a hormonal change, and just like it did at puberty, your body adapts. You're still you. You go back to who you were before the change."

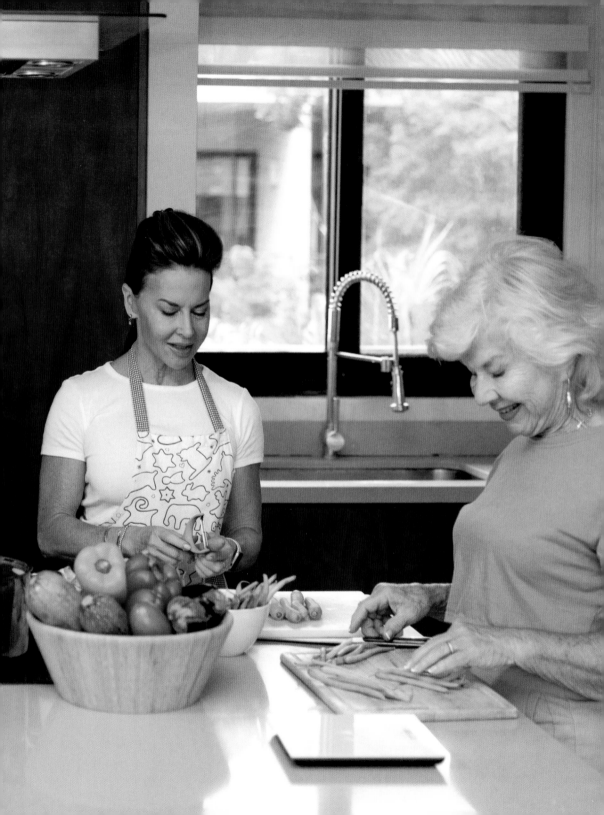

FINDING WHAT WORKS FOR YOU

No program is one-size-fits-all and the important thing is to start with the premise that you're worth it. This is your moment, your hour, your year. The program posits small, regular meals at three-hour intervals. What if you work in an office? Making it work for you might involve spending time at home creating meals you can take with you and pop in your work refrigerator. If you're a morning person, do your cardio first thing in the morning and feel the energy all day. Night owl? Work out in the evening with your workday behind you.

Change will only work if it doesn't become, well, unworkable. And you've probably already experienced the need to work around some of the nonnegotiables in your life. If you know you're no good in the mornings, you probably don't schedule important meetings then, right? You create a schedule you can live with. Making change doesn't have to turn your world completely upside down, although, in time, you might find that it does—and welcome the disruption!

PREPARING YOURSELF FOR CHANGE

Transformation doesn't happen overnight and it doesn't happen without intention. And while your family doesn't need to be 100% on board with the transformations you're prepared to make, they need to know that change is on the way.

Individuals and families fall into habits—some of which are healthy and some of which aren't. The challenge here is to understand that you'll be letting go of some things. You'll replace them with better, clearer, healthier habits, but it's important to not minimize the loss. As you examine what you're doing now, you'll probably find that some of your habits aren't in your best interests. They aren't truly working *for* you. You might be accustomed to eating dinner in front of the TV in record time, but if you take a step back and really think about that practice, you'll probably agree it doesn't bring out the best in you, your food, or even your TV viewing.

Thinking through some of the ways your daily routines and attitudes need to change will help when it actually comes to making those choices reality. How do you cope with stress? Do you reach for a cookie or a glass of wine? How do you deal with long hours in front of a computer?

Imagining yourself in various ordinary situations and visualizing making healthier choices around them will help prepare you for those moments and decisions when they become real. Imagine ducking out for a quick walk around the block when you've been sitting at your desk for a couple hours instead of heading for the refrigerator. Imagine feeling stress building up and doing some stretching and deep breathing instead of pouring that automatic glass of wine. See yourself doing different, healthy things in response to the challenges of everyday life. Spend time with those images. Call them to mind frequently.

If you can visualize yourself being an active, healthy, fulfilled individual, you're closer to becoming that person.

"I don't think I was always aware I was making choices," says Joan. "I just did things on automatic pilot. Sometimes, I did the same things I'd always done only because I never questioned them. I learned from my parents how to be an adult—and that's the adult I became."

Stepping back from automatic pilot allows you to see who's really in the driver's seat. Is it the child whose decisions were made for her or the adult who's taking her time over her choices? "You can pick a whole different life for yourself as an adult with your adult wisdom," says Joan.

That "adult wisdom" doesn't need to extinguish childlike enthusiasm. "It's about tapping into the same freedom you used to allow yourself," says Joan. "Think about combining the imagination of a child with the wisdom of an adult! What we're doing is changing our bodies—and the mind is along for the ride. Remember when you used to think 'I can do my own thing'? So do it now!"

UNDERSTANDING PLANNING

Accept that planning is going to be a major part of your life going forward. It's obvious we don't control everything in our lives: The unexpected happens, people take actions that impact our lives, the weather changes. But there's a difference between allowing for plans to change and not making plans at all!

We'll be going into some detail about meal planning and workout planning later in the book, but for now, let's look at why that's going to be helpful.

The advantages to planning your meals might seem obvious, but there are hidden surprises and gains you might not have considered. Preplanned meals, especially those created by a nutritionist, have more fiber and vegetables, fewer carbohydrates, and less sodium, sugar, and saturated fat than meals you might make up on the fly or eat at a restaurant. Preplanning (and sticking to your plan!) increases your probability of reaching all your health goals: losing weight, improving your heart health, and keeping your blood sugar in check. Meal planning is what gives you ingredients and resources to actually make this happen on a daily basis.

"It's all about preparation!" says Joan. "Even when you travel—and I travel a lot—you can plan. Look at where you're going and what you'll be doing. I often bring something in a container that doesn't need to be heated. As long as you work your meals around your macros, you can make it work. You just have to be thoughtful. There's protein powder with coconut milk. Good-quality protein bars with not as many carbs. There are products you can use if you need to. The most important thing is to fit your meals into your plan. I even have a food scale that folds up to make it easier to pack. You can get through anything with some planning ahead of time."

Meal planning is associated with increased food variety—a key component of a healthy diet that increases the likelihood of meeting nutrient needs and making healthy eating a lot less dull. Perhaps even more importantly, cooking at home also gives you control and choice over ingredients.

Likewise, planning your workout routine means you're far more likely to stick to it. Thinking "I might go to the gym this afternoon" is a far cry from "I'm going to go do my workout at 3 p.m." Preplanning means being organized so you don't realize at the last minute that you have an important telephone call to make or that your workout clothes are all in the wash or that you forgot to get gas for the car so you can get to the fitness center.

HOW TO GET STARTED

Success in this next chapter of your life is more assured the more prepared you are. There are plans to be created, actions to be taken, purchases to be made. And, of course, a mindset to be developed!

You aren't going to magically get more active overnight. Think about what you need in order to get going: You have to get ready to be more active and more mindful of your eating habits.

We've already talked about preparing your mindset, but you also need to think about what you need to tuck into your budget going forward, such as exercise clothes, weights, a gym membership, hiring a personal trainer and/or nutritionist.

In terms of practicality, you'll need some items to get started:

- Tape measure

- Scale for weighing yourself

- Scale for weighing your food

- Workout clothes (including several pairs of sneakers)

- Access to a gym or fitness club and/or weights at home

- Access to the internet

- Smartphone/tablet app to keep track of progress and/or a journal in which to record nutrition and workouts

Joan says she finds the last item on the list the most difficult to master. "Even after all this time, I'm not terribly technical!" she laments. "But I stick to it."

Eventually, as you begin lifting more weight, you'll want to buy a weight belt that will support your back and keep you from injuring yourself.

Also, get ready to change your outlook. One of the books Michelle recommends is *Think Like a Warrior* by Darrin Donnelly. While its examples aren't within everyone's experience, expertise, or area of interest—it draws on lessons learned and taught by professional sports coaches—its message is for everyone.

In fact, "reading can be a great way to bolster your mindset, take a few minutes out of your day to relax, and educate yourself on new material so you can keep working on your personal growth and development," says Michelle. Other titles she recommends include James Clear's *Atomic Habits*, Kathryn Hanson's *Brain Over Binge*, Miguel Ruiz's *The Four Agreements*, Gay Hendrix's *The Big Leap*, and Donnelly's *Relentless Optimism*.

Deb Black

The Wonder Women transformation program is a gift of self-love. I'm humbled, honored, and filled with gratitude to have been a part of it. It all started when I viewed a clip of Joan MacDonald's transformation in her 70s. I was blown away by her success. What a wonderful life this woman is living!

And so it began. I emptied my soul into my application—and acceptance into the program was such an emotional moment for me. Life is always about timing. I wasn't sure what I'd be capable of, but clearly, Michelle was. Her accomplishments personally and professionally speak volumes about who she is and how well she knows the female anatomy. I was 69 when I started The Wonder Women, the oldest in my group, with too many injuries to mention.

Michelle treats all her clients in the same unique way. Age is irrelevant. We all chop wood and carry water, count macros, train, drink lots of water, rest, and reflect on what we need to do to reach our goals. The mindset part of the program demanded we dig deep every day, peel away the layers of doubt, explore new possibilities, create daily habits, break down barriers, and learn to say no. It took some time and tough love from Michelle and weekly check-in photos—they were all the motivation I needed to fuel the fire.

I'm part of a Tribe of Women who support each other completely. We're worldwide and come from all walks of life. We stumble, we learn, we grow, we heal, and we continue to transform. We're living our best lives. I'm a powerhouse, ready to start each day with wisdom, purpose, joy, and gratitude.

There are no words that could thank Michelle and Joan for sharing their knowledge, kindness, and courage with the world. They're exceptional role models who work tirelessly to help women transform. They're loved by all who embrace them. I'll continue to shine brightly for all the work they've put into me and live an exceptional life, as they do. To the women unsure of taking the big leap: Jump right in—the water's perfect in the Wonder Women Sea!

CHAPTER FOUR:

FITNESS FUNDAMENTALS

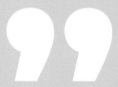

The point of the physical journey is to truly know yourself and guide yourself with wisdom and clarity.

Michelle MacDonald

The statistic is sobering: Only 23% of adults aged 18 and above meet the recommended guidelines for aerobic and muscle-strengthening activity. The biggest hurdle for most people is—theoretically at least—not having enough time. But a 2019 study from the Centers for Disease Control and Prevention and the Rand Corporation, surveying more than 30,000 participants, found that Americans have an average of more than 5 hours of free time per day.

So there's definitely time to work out. There's time to build muscle and endurance and find a fitness level you might have only dreamed of in the past.

When we think about "fitness," we often focus on aesthetics. We imagine being able to wear a bikini. But fitness is first and foremost about health.

As a society, our lifestyle choices and stress management techniques (such as they are) have created an epidemic of hypertension. Hypertension—or, as it's known more colloquially, high blood pressure—is the pressure of blood on the walls of the arteries carrying blood from our hearts to the rest of our bodies. Blood pressure goes up and down throughout the day—trending lower when we're relaxed and resting; higher when we're stressed and anxious or in pain. When blood pressure remains high for an extended period of time, it puts us at risk for strokes, heart attacks, and other major health threats because our organs aren't absorbing the blood they need.

Other risks posed by sedentary lives include such chronic conditions as type 2 diabetes, heart disease, many types of cancer, depression and anxiety, and dementia.

BUILDING MUSCLE
IS FUNDAMENTAL

Muscle is the organ of longevity. There's robust research showing that more muscle mass will help you better handle disease, stress, illness, and injury at all stages of life—but especially as you age.

"Build muscle!" exclaims Michelle. "A good amount of quality muscle on your body will improve insulin sensitivity, improve blood sugar control, and reduce the likelihood of falls by improving balance and fortifying bones, ligaments, and tendons. It will also improve your sleep and mental health, and it's directly linked to longevity."

Lack of muscle is directly linked to age-related problems. For example, you might have heard of sarcopenia, an age-related, involuntary loss of skeletal muscle mass and strength. It doesn't just affect older adults either; sarcopenia can begin in your 40s—and some people lose up to 50% of their muscle mass by the time they're in their 80s.

That's the bad news. The good news? "Sarcopenia is reversible with just a couple days of weight training," says Michelle. "What we call 'normal aging' is actually what we'd associate with lifestyle issues that don't support muscle growth."

In other words, our culture has taken a preventable problem and normalized it to the point of expectation. Muscle growth and maintenance are available to you and will help you stay healthy and vital no matter what your age. We tend to associate the thought of building muscle with athletes in training—necessary for young people on sports teams or running races. But older people need muscle growth as much as—if not more than—younger people.

In fact, muscle growth is especially important to older adults. For example, 1 in 3 women and 1 in 12 men will sustain a hip fracture in their lifetime, with 86% of hip fractures occurring in individuals 65 and older. Hip fractures are associated with significant morbidity, mortality, loss of independence, and financial burden.

"Fast-twitch muscles are the powerful ones," says Michelle. "Fast-twitch muscles aren't good for endurance, but they're excellent for reflexes—they're what will help you catch yourself from a fall." Fast-twitch muscles support short, quick bursts of energy—the kind you need for sprinting or powerlifting. But they're also the muscles that respond quickly to events outside the body, including a loss of balance.

Building fast-twitch muscles through weight training, along with consuming enough calories to support bone density, can reduce rates of falling and subsequent fractures—and that alone might make the practice worthwhile!

As we'll see, part of building muscle is doing it through a program that allows you to track your progress on a daily basis. "Before I started the transformation program, I never journaled, never took regular body measurements or photos to see how I was doing," says Joan. "I never consistently managed my nutrition or trained using a training log. Like most other people, I didn't realize there was an entire system out there that anyone can follow."

BUILDING MUSCLE IN YOUR BODY

Building muscle isn't just about health and vitality—it's also about aesthetics. "Muscle lies on top of bone and under skin," says Michelle. "That's where fat is too. But muscle has shape, whereas fat doesn't. Fat has no tone, so it falls and sags. So an older body with muscle looks completely different from a body that doesn't have muscle. The truth is, things fall south, but that has more to do with lifestyle than with age."

Most women focus on cardiovascular workouts and neglect weight training. "When you think of the gym, you think of cardio," says Michelle. "Women aren't really encouraged to go and lift weights. Most fitness centers aren't about lifting. But that's what's going to build muscle—and so much more."

Women need strength training, endurance training, and a solid nutrition plan. They all work together. The combination provides a number of health benefits: increasing longevity, decreasing osteoporosis, improving sleep, regulating moods, and even improving digestion. "I really feel a lot younger than I did before," says Joan. "I used to take all kinds of medications that I don't need now."

Building muscle also means you can—and should—eat more to feed your effort. "Women start out the program eating like birds because that's what diets tell them to do," says Michelle. "And by the end, they're eating as much as their sons in college are. And you have to ask 'How come we didn't know about this?' It's so huge and that message isn't getting out. It's an easy fix. You're not preparing for

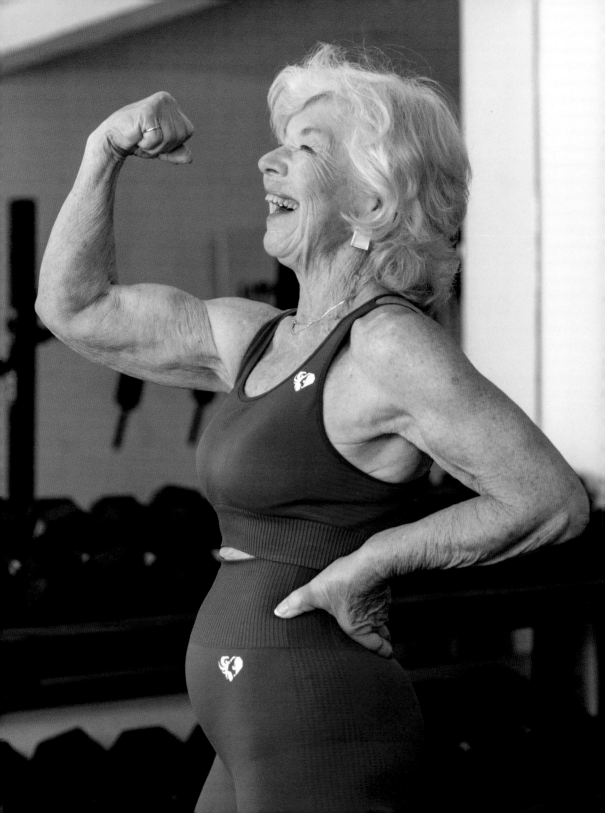

a bodybuilding show. All you have to do is commit six months to a year. You'll lose 20 to 30 pounds with 3 to 7 months of work, then rebuild your body the way you want it after the weight loss. That's such a small investment for the amount of benefits you'll have forever!"

Michelle really does means forever. "If you pursue building muscle as you age, you'll live longer and better," she says. "You'll have a healthier lifestyle, plus the great emotional side effects you get from all those endorphins!"

BUILDING MUSCLE SAFELY

Michelle's advice: "Go nice and slow. Don't move slowly, but work your way into your program slowly," she says. It's important to consult your health care provider and get a physical/medical examination before starting an exercise routine. This is particularly important if you're new to strenuous and vigorous physical activities.

An early checkup can detect any health problems or conditions that could put you at risk for an injury during exercise. It can also help you optimize your workout, making it easier for you and your personal trainer—should you choose to work with one—to understand what limitations you might have and create an exercise plan that suits and supports your particular needs. "It's not complicated," says Michelle. "The human body is pretty basic. The body responds to the same pressures. You need to think about medical considerations but also your athletic abilities. Someone might be able to do a squat, whereas someone else could substitute a leg press instead."

If you're unsure of your health status, have known health problems, or are pregnant, speak with your doctor before starting your program.

"Make sure it's okay to work out," says Michelle. "And ask what you need to stay away from even inside your exercise program. For example, if you have high blood pressure, you can't do sprints until it comes down. And make sure you're following a program you can sustain. Building muscle requires consistency in your exercise routine as well as your nutrition so you can support muscle protein synthesis."

For added safety, ask a professional trainer to help you put your program together. They'll teach you the correct form to use for every different exercise so you don't inadvertently injure yourself.

FINDING AN EXPERT GUIDE

In fact, relying on professionals—experts—is what will make your fitness routines safe and effective.

But first, it's worth noting we've been using the terms "coach" and "trainer" pretty much interchangeably. There are a few key differences between them, although the experience with each might feel similar.

Coaches are mentors who understand their clients' specific physical, emotional, and dietary needs, limitations, and desires. They work with their clients to develop goals, enabling them to live healthy, vital lives.

Personal trainers have historically focused on the exercise part of their clients' fitness journeys, helping create workout plans and routines to help achieve a client's goals. Trainers might assist with nutrition if they have the proper background and certification, but their primary focus is on the exercise side of things. Coaching tends to be longer term than training, as it's learning about how to live rather than just how to exercise.

"A great coach should not only have the knowledge necessary to teach you how to do something, but they should also have faith in you. They should believe you can accomplish it," says Joan. "A great coach can envision your possibilities before you can see them yourself."

A personal trainer or coach is someone who'll be good at "putting you through your paces," as Joan says. "A coach can improve your game. A great coach can change your life." And in fact, when you share your needs and goals with your coach, you're tackling any number of issues: family, work, health, pleasures. "I take notes on everything," says Michelle. "What's your internal narrative? Are you feeding your focus—or are you feeding your fears?"

Choosing between a coach and a personal trainer depends on a number of factors, including geography, cost, availability, and more. The title is less important than what they have to offer and whether that syncs with what you need.

When you're searching for a trainer, look for someone with accreditation in good standing with a national certification board. While there are any number of them available, the following have the best governing boards:

- The **International Sports Sciences Association (ISSA)** bills itself as "the trainer's trainer," offering a variety of self-paced distance courses on many different fitness and health-related topics.

- The **National Council on Strength & Fitness (NCSF)** is a globally recognized organization for exercise professionals, accredited in the United States (NCCA) and Europe (EA) and offering certification at more than 1,000 testing sites in 83 countries.

Exercise professionals can specialize in personal training, strength and conditioning, and sports and fitness nutrition.

- The **National Strength and Conditioning Association (NSCA)** offers industry-leading certifications, research journals, career development services, networking opportunities, and continuing education. The organization includes 60,000 researchers, educators, strength and conditioning coaches, performance and sport scientists, personal trainers, tactical professionals, and other related roles.

- The **American Council on Exercise (ACE)** focuses on training courses and resources accredited by the National Commission for Certifying Agencies (NCCA), with certifications in personal training, health coaching, fitness instruction, and medical exercise specializations.

- The **National Academy of Sports Medicine (NASM)** offers an elite, science-based approach to personal training that includes certifications in sports nutrition, personal training, and general wellness coaching.

Beyond accreditation, Michelle recommends checking with your potential trainer for case studies and references. "In the modern era, with social media, there should be at least five people in your demographic they can give for references. They should be proud to do that. Otherwise, continue looking!"

Your potential trainer should also be happy to be interviewed. "The trainer should be excited to work with you," says Michelle. "They should ask you a lot of questions about your personal life and put together a program that's specifically for you and your needs. It's not one-size-fits-all. Plans should take medications, goals, your current fitness level, all that into consideration. There should always be good communication between you and your trainer. Ask them to show you how they'd put your program together before signing on."

That said, using a trainer doesn't have to last forever. For many people, the cost becomes an issue—and that shouldn't stand in the way. "You don't have to spend tons and tons of money. You just want to be very organized. If you're not good at correcting and so on, then invest in a trainer and a coach. If you have the budget for it, it will save you time," says Michelle. "But you can also hire a trainer for the first week or two, then by and large, you're good to go on your own. Just make an appointment to brush up later. That's the most cost-effective way to do it. There are so many videos online that will help you with your form once you have your training plan in place. Watch for the ones that have had the most views. That generally means they're going to be helpful."

CHOOSING THE ROUTINES YOU NEED

When you're starting out, be conscious of doing a program you can do consistently. Can you realistically commit to working out five days a week? How about three days? Talk with your trainer to set up a program you can actually follow.

Having a way of keeping track (more on this later) will help in tweaking your routine and improving your form. "Do a video of yourself," says Joan. "You'll be able to see things you miss when you're just looking in the mirror."

Michelle is constantly underlining consistency. "You need to follow a program appropriate to your abilities," she says. "Hire someone, do it on an app, just make sure you do something that's planned and thought through. Most gyms have a trainer who'll walk you through the equipment use and show you how to lift properly. Then, after that, you can watch videos and watch other people at the gym to make sure your form is correct."

Joan adds: "Feel free to ask people for help. Most people are happy to. When you go to the gym, if you do it at the same time every day, chances are you'll keep seeing the same people. And they'll keep seeing you. I've had young guys come up to me and comment on my progress. And that makes me feel like I can ask them for tips when I need to. There's a lot of respect for each other."

"Make sure you always record what you do," says Michelle. "Keep track of the weight you lift and the number of weights you do. And just understand that the first week, you're going to be sore!"

Another term that comes up along with consistency is "progressive change." "Your first week, you want to go on the lighter side, take notes, and each week go a little heavier," Michelle explains. "Keep focusing on your form. Once your form is good, either add weight or add reps." This technique is called "progressive overload." "Make it harder every week, forcing your body to adapt. The body heals and adapts, so what was hard becomes easy."

In the simplest terms, progressive overload does mean lifting heavier weights each and every workout. But depending on your program, you can focus on other ways of creating a progressive overload for your body. You can increase your training frequency, doing more

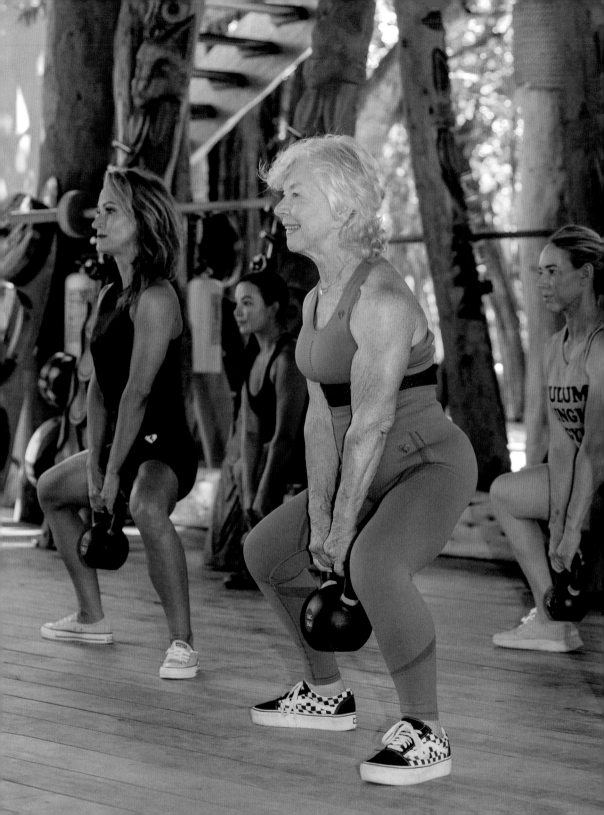

training or focusing on a specific body part more frequently during the week. Or you can focus on more range of motion—for example, making your squats a little deeper each workout. You can also consider training intensity by keeping track of how elevated your heart rate is and for how long or training density by pushing yourself to do more training in the same time frame.

So as you establish your routine, remember that it's not always about lifting heavier weights. "Before you increase, you have to improve your form," says Michelle. "It's very common for beginners to have poor motor patterning, so it doesn't serve them to add weight because then you cement bad habits." The better the technique, the better your muscle recruitment.

She recommends constantly checking posture. "Older clients usually have poor glute mechanics," she says. "You have to get the process down: Stabilize yourself, then transfer the force from your lower body to your upper body. A lot of people don't activate their glutes very well." Poor glute mechanics can lead to or exacerbate the knee issues common in older adults.

There are a number of areas Joan and Michelle focus on that aren't typically given a lot of attention. For example, you might not have heard of the transverse abdominis (TVA) muscle, but it's one of your best friends: It acts as a stabilizer for your lower back and core muscles. "Your TVA muscles are stretched in obesity and childbirth," says Michelle. "Working your abs will strengthen your TVA. There's a lot that can be healed and reversed—but people don't know about it. For women, pelvic floor health is huge. Incontinence in older women isn't de rigueur. You really can heal your pelvic floor."

She's passionate about women becoming better educated about their bodies, particularly as they age. "I want to help as many women as I can to take back their health," Michelle says. "Ever since the 1950s, there's been this marketing push that pathologizes hormonal cycles, conception, and menopause. Women get strung out on steroids and drugs. They get prescribed medications for everything—anxiety, insomnia, weight gain. There's a whole industry dedicated to making women feel sick. And no one talks about it."

Michelle and Joan—and the many women who are part of their programs or follow them on social media—are out to change that. To talk about it. To learn from each other. "The way women are marketed to in the United States is significantly different from Germany or France," says Michelle. "The American market is number one in the world for prescription opiates. Think about that. The most powerful nation in the world is strung out as a population."

And they don't need to be. While Michelle confesses herself as being "on the fence" about hormone replacement therapy (HRT), she doesn't ever see it as a first response. "Lifestyle changes can do just as good a job. If you work out, if you explore a new way of eating, if you're drinking enough water, you don't experience all the negative effects of menopause. HRT is pushed a little too hard. It's not the magical fountain of youth. Your mindset, your internal dialogue—that's what makes the difference."

Michelle's advice? "Get your blood work done. Find an endocrinologist who specializes in menopause," she says. "Just treat doctors like any other professional!"

RECORD EVERYTHING

Keeping track of what you're doing is essential to your success. Going to a gym without a fitness journal is like going on a journey without GPS or a map—you might sort of remember where you've been, you might know where you're heading, but you don't know exactly how to get there. And there's a good chance you'll waste a lot of effort along the way.

You can do it the low-tech way: keeping a notebook in which you write down your daily weight training (specific body part being worked, weights, and the number of repetitions), your cardiovascular workouts (exercises, duration, heart rate, and specific cardio equipment), even your steps.

It can also be helpful to record other details: how much sleep you got or didn't experience the night before, your motivations, your current mood, your energy levels. And, of course, record your weight and measurements on a regular basis.

The Train with Joan app is one of the best available. It gives you workouts to follow, spaces to log your progress, and a community with which to share your journey.

WHAT'S IT LIKE TO WORK OUT?

Joan and Michelle agree that workouts should be tailored to your specific needs, goals, and abilities. "Everyone does it differently," says Joan. "Michelle says a good workout can be done in an hour, although I've never managed that. Mine are an hour and a half to two hours. I'm slow! But you also have to let your muscles adjust to what you're doing with them. It's a lot of time out of the day, but once you get into the rhythm, it's not a big thing. Mostly I'm still sorting out the times when I should be doing and when I should be resting."

Part of the challenge is the shared space in a gym. "It's not fair in a busy gym to linger around a machine," says Joan. "That happens so much. Some people don't have the concept of sharing. And a lot of people are in the gym way longer than they need to be."

People go to gyms for a number of different reasons. What's important is for you to be clear on what yours are and not get derailed comparing yourself with anyone else.

"At first, I worried that others were judging me, especially the men," says Joan. "But after a while, you don't notice them as much because you're focused. And after they've seen you for a while, they respect what you're doing. Most of the men are complimentary. They notice when you're making progress or they'll tell you if you're doing something that could injure you. They'll step in and offer alternatives. That's really helpful. My son-in-law does that for me too: If I say this exercise hurts too much, he'll give me an alternative."

And it works both ways. "In between sets, I might let my eyes wander, and if I see someone struggling, I might make a suggestion, but I don't stare at them. True gym rats are concentrating on themselves, not on anyone else," Joan says.

She goes in prepared. "I always have a list of the exercises I'm going to do during a workout," Joan says. "I love listening to music—I like mellow country, classical, blues, jazz, even rock and roll—but sometimes, it's more of a distraction than a help. And besides, I want to do my exercises concisely so they don't drag on and music can make me forget my time. What I really want to take on is the mental challenge of taking a couple minutes off the time, not add to it!"

There's no magic formula for the perfect workout. You do your reps, drink your water, watch your form, record your work. "Just be mindful of how many sets and reps you have to do for a given exercise," counsels Joan. "Ask yourself: 'What did I do the last time and can I improve on it? Can I add more weight? How about more reps?'"

If you have a good fitness plan, there's plenty of variety in your daily regimen. "I do shoulders and arms on one day. Another day, I'll do my chest and back, and all I really think about is how many sets, reps, what's the rest time in between, and can I improve my time," says Joan.

HOW TO HANDLE DISRUPTIONS

They'll happen. No matter what you do, your routine *will* be disrupted at many points along the journey. You can't control the world. You can't control other people. Accepting that disruptions will come your way is the best first step in handling them.

Michelle advises: "Be historical. We tend to repeat the same cycles over and over again. See how you handled disruptions in the past and learn from that."

Joan and Michelle believe strongly in keeping records. "Journals provide that aha moment," says Joan.

"You get better at having a grounding discussion with yourself," says Michelle. "Imagine you're talking with your best friend. How would you encourage them? You don't tell them they're a failure. What have they done right? That outweighs anything disrupting."

If you miss a workout because of a situation beyond your control, allow yourself to feel the pain of missing something, but don't let it dictate your future. "We all have old programming," says Michelle. "For example, in the past, you might have said 'I always screw up when I'm stressed'. But keeping the journal shows the times you've been stressed and you haven't screwed up. And there will be more and more of them."

Keep lists. "Keep a list of ideas that work and another list of ideas that didn't work," says Michelle. "Like substituting a brisk walk when you can't make it to the gym—that's an idea that works. On the other hand, going out to dinner and just winging it might not have worked so well. Remind yourself of both. By three months in, you'll pretty much know what will and won't work for you."

You can also plan for disruptions. You might not know specifically what disruption will occur, but knowing they're inevitable, you can prepare. Joan and Michelle recommend recording a "rainy day video" for yourself and have it ready to view on the day you need it—when you've had a disruption to your routine: *Hey, girl, you just got a little lost. This is what I need you to do now.* ...

Creating this personalized video will help you get back to where you need to be. "Leave yourself messages so you can talk yourself off the ledge," says Michelle. "Have a whole toolkit that keeps you on the winning side of things."

The more you record, the stronger you'll be because your journal can also be a historical record. It enables you to go back and derive strength from those things that have worked for you in the past and avoid some of the pitfalls you've encountered. "If you can learn to go back again and again, you can trace the pattern of your success," says Michelle. "You already have a history of what did and didn't work. If you do that enough times, you'll remove yourself quickly from the pattern of failure."

"Let's look at it from a coach's perspective," she says. "Look at your comparison photos. Look at the data and facts. You've been at it 2 months. You've lost 6 inches and 12 pounds. You've done the mindset work, you've figured out your triggers, you're able to do critical thinking fast, you're self-aware. Looking at it that way, your disruption is just a drop in the bucket. The perspective is huge."

FITNESS & MOTIVATION (AGAIN!)

"You know, when I don't feel like working out—those feelings are fleeting," says Joan. "Once I get to the gym and do my warmups, I'm fine. It changes my whole persona. It's like getting dressed: If you only get half-dressed, you're vulnerable. You feel something's incomplete. If I didn't work out, I'd feel a big part of my life was missing."

It's been that way for her almost since the start. "My worst problems with motivation were during the first year," she says. "That was when I sometimes wanted to throw the towel in. I wanted to be done. I didn't realize there *is* no 'done.' It's a change you make to your whole life. It's just how you do things."

Joan gets a lot of her fitness motivation from her daughter. "Even when Michelle isn't feeling well or has an injury, she'll still do some sort of exercise. It's her lifestyle. Think of it this way: It's an honor to be able to do it. When you can live a better life, it's an honor for you to look after your body because it's what's going to carry you through. And it affects everything: how you feel about yourself, how you start every morning, how peaceful you feel when you go to bed at night."

Committing to a fitness routine can go far beyond the physical. "It's a great platform for transforming your whole life," says Michelle. "Before Mom started, she was angry, frustrated, depressed. What I saw was that she was heading nowhere fast. Now she's excited. She used to snap at things. Now she doesn't. She hugs. She's happy."

"It's kind of like growing up," says Joan. "When you're a kid, you can't wait until you're older. Then you get to be an adult, and you think 'Oh no, now I have to parent myself!' And you get overwhelmed—whether it's your health or your finances or your relationships—but when you journal and practice meditation and work on things that are difficult, you change internally. And you see that now you're an adult, anything is truly possible. If you change the way you perceive the world, the world actually changes. It's that dramatic. It's not anything woo-woo. It's basic. You have to learn to be the hero of your own movie. You don't want to be just that other character."

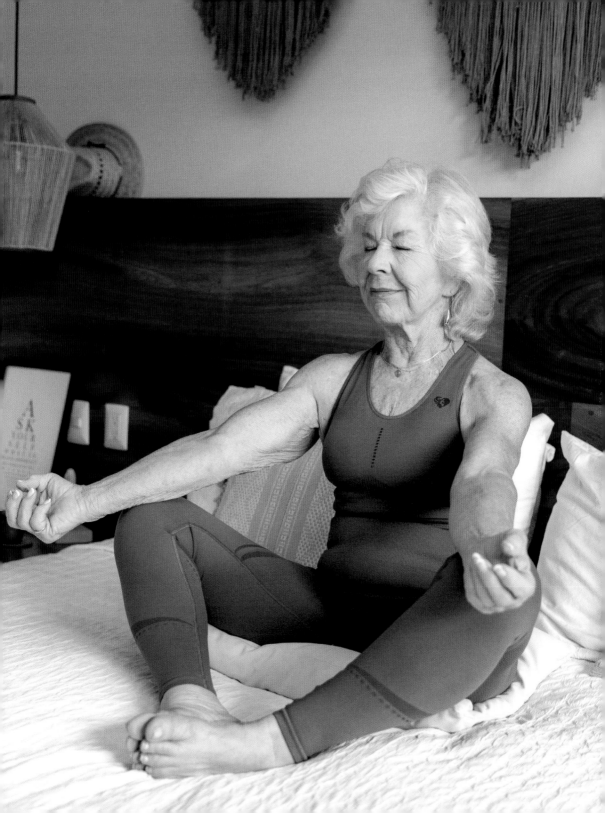

Trish Cheatham

As a busy CEO and single mom of an autistic child, I led an extremely stressful life and was always on the go. I put other people's needs ahead of my own and felt I never had time to take care of me. I've been fit most of my life but lost myself somewhere along the way with all the overwhelming stress I was dealing with. I truly didn't realize how much weight I'd gained until I became very ill in February 2022 and ended up in the ER, unable to breathe.

While in the ER, the doctor told me I was over 200 pounds and that my blood pressure was so high, I could have a stroke at any moment. In that instant, I was terrified— all I could think about was what would happen if I died and left my son alone with no one to take care of him?

In that moment, I begged God to let me live so I could take care of my child and I vowed to do whatever it took to get healthy and to take better care of myself. I remembered running across Joan's Instagram account at work one day and showing my staff her page. "Look at this woman!" If a 70-year-old Joan could transform like that, I knew I could too. I started researching Joan and ran across her daughter Michelle's program and applied, all while starting to eat healthy on my own and moving my body—keeping that promise I made to myself and God.

By this time, COVID had struck and we were in lockdown. I figured if we had to be in lockdown, it might as well be someplace interesting, so I bought an Airstream trailer and my son, my fiancé, and our dogs took off for a trip across the United States, living in the Airstream for months.

Before we set off, I got the news I'd been selected for Michelle's program. When I told her I'd be doing the program on the road, I know she immediately thought, "Well, this one won't make it!." But I was determined. I loaded up our rig with all I would need—adjustable weights, bands, straps, sandbags, and more—and we set off on our adventure.

Unfortunately, the Airstream's electrical blew up at our first stop. My fiancé was working hard to fix the problem and we didn't know if we could continue on our trip. But I still had a workout to do. So off I went—outside the Airstream, working out, sweating, sobbing uncontrollably— so worried. I sent my workout video to Michelle, who didn't mention my crying and critiqued my form. I thought to myself, "Does she even care?" But in that moment, I vowed to myself I would never quit. I'd always show up for myself and prove to my coach I was worthy to be there. I made sure I never, ever had an excuse.

My journey showed me it was okay to put myself first. That by putting myself first I was better able to take care of my family, my child, my employees, and my clients. I'm a better person for everyone when I take care of myself—clearer and so much more energy. It was fascinating to watch people around me become happier because I was happier.

I tell women constantly that if I can do this, you can too. I'm not special. I'm just someone who made a promise to myself and never gave up. I never made one excuse. I never stopped. And because of that, I now have the most incredible life and I'm able to experience the most amazing joys with my son. And THAT is the greatest gift of all.

CHAPTER FIVE:

NUTRITION FUNDAMENTALS

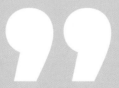

I'm really glad Michelle figured all this stuff out for me. It's obvious after you've been following it for a while that it really is easy to do, but someone had to do it first. And now, like they say, there's an app for that!

Joan MacDonald

There are a lot of ways to lose weight. There are a lot of ways to keep weight off. Some are more successful than others. The trouble is, it's difficult to find a nutrition program that does both. Macro-based eating does just that—and fuels your body appropriately for whatever challenges you encounter (or make for yourself) in life. Macro-based meal planning and nutrition allow you to have agency to make food choices, restore vitality, and give your body exactly what it needs.

Why does a macro-based diet make a difference? For one thing, it's all about choices you can make. "Everyone can prioritize what they're eating according to their taste," says Michelle. "There's so much autonomy in crafting sustainable, delicious meals. What one person eats won't look at all like what someone else eats. And it allows you to continue to evolve with new ingredients and recipes, which has the result of making it much more sustainable." For example: "If you really want ice cream or chocolate, you can find a way to fit it in."

Diets have traditionally been binary: This food is good; that food isn't. Only eat from this category; never eat from that one. "Think of your diet plan as a budget," Michelle says. "If you're clever, you can have fun with the plan and live happily ever after. Getting weight off has never been the problem. It's keeping it off. Eighty percent of people who've lost weight on a diet regain that weight in the first year. That's huge! The problem has always been sustainability."

This is a big step away from how most women were introduced to dieting. Diets traditionally restrict calories until a weight goal has been attained, but no one can stay on a diet forever, always wishing they could eat beloved and forbidden foods and essentially waiting to get "off" the diet so they can go back to them. There's something inherently judgmental and punitive about plans that make women constantly suppress their appetites and deny themselves foods they love. On the other hand, macro-based nutrition plans encourage satiation and enable women to eat their favorite foods in balance with others.

One way of looking at it is this: Macros are your food calories organized into nutrient groups: protein, fat, and carbs. Each of these groups provides different health benefits that work together to keep you vital and healthy. Counting macros won't just help you lose weight. It can help control your appetite, support your energy, and protect your lean mass. You can lose more fat, build more muscle, and achieve better overall results with a macro-based nutrition program as compared with a calorie-controlled diet.

As we'll see, there are some calculations required for this plan— and that's not a bad thing. It gives participants a certain freedom. "Women can think of food differently," says Michelle. "Instead of just thinking tasty stuff, they can see food has a mathematical value structure." This takes food out of the realm of feelings and puts it squarely in the realm of reality.

Overall, "psychologically, calculating your macros makes a difference," says Michelle. "Take the time to understand what makes you hungry or full. You really get to know yourself. And making your own plan is so empowering. It gives back the power that binary diets take away. It just bypasses any resistance women have to a cookie-cutter plan. And that means it can also encompass different cultures, which is also huge."

It's also an important way for older women to look at what they're eating and what they can expect to achieve. "Equations are typically based on estimates that might not be reflective of the person you're talking to," says Michelle. "They're based on college boys. There's a narrative out there that says females change after menopause—that it's inevitable for them to acquire that midsection, that belly. Suck it up, cupcake. There hasn't been a lot of support for women who are seeking and experiencing a different outcome."

"Older women don't love their bodies," she adds. "But they could."

INTRODUCTION TO MACRO-BASED EATING

The first thing you need to know about following Michelle and Joan's prescription for healthy eating is this: It looks complicated. And it might feel that way at the start. But as with any habit, once you start practicing it, then over time, it gets to be second nature.

The second thing you need to understand is this: You're going to have to convert your thinking from the imperial system of weights and measurements to the metric one. It's easier to calculate and it's a great deal more precise. "Why grams? Professional kitchens use grams—and we're aiming for that same precision," says Michelle. "There's a high degree of accuracy and you can scale it, which is hard to do in the imperial system."

Let's start with the basics: Everything we eat is a collection of macronutrients. They're what our bodies require to be nourished and function. You might not be consciously aware of what they're called or what roles they play, but you already consume macronutrients in the proteins, fats, and carbohydrates you eat every day. And your body requires all three. No diet should keep you from eating any of them because they're the nutritive components of food your body needs for energy and to maintain its structure and systems.

There are many different ways to approach nutrition. Joan's program uses a macro-based approach in which target protein, carbohydrate, and fat intake per meal are determined. This is quite different from the typical "calories per day" approach used by many diets—and, to be frank, by many medical and fitness professionals still grounded in that seemingly immutable mindset.

"It means you'll get exactly what your body needs right now—no more and no less," says Joan.

Instead of employing a "calories per day" strategy, this approach determines and follows individual macro goals on a daily basis and dispenses them in a balanced manner over the course of five or six meals. That means you're supporting your body regularly with food and therefore avoiding the highs and lows of so-called "yo-yo" dieting. It's a sustainable approach that won't just help you with body transformation but will also allow you to maintain your physique no matter what age you are. "We don't tell clients what to eat," says Michelle. "They have the flexibility to create their own meals within the macro goals tailored for them, their body type, and their physique goals. It's essential for long-term success and balance."

But there's a caveat: "It's a misconception to think that the key to weight loss or transformation comes down to having the perfect plan or knowing what macros to follow," says Michelle. "If that were true, then everyone who had a program written out for them would be successful—and that's simply not the case.

"Knowing what macros to follow isn't the key to success. The key to success is being the person who follows the plan. Like everything else external, macros are simply tools."

Having the right tool is fine, but using the right tool is what matters most. "People who are successful at anything are successful first and foremost because they have the right mindset," says Michelle. "They'd be successful at any plan you give them because that's just how their brain is wired."

Every food has calories. They're not going to magically disappear just because you're looking at them differently. But those calories can be used in different and more interesting ways. "I just divide my meal up into proteins, carbs, and fats," says Joan. "Then I can create whatever meal I want!"

"Be proud of being clever," urges Michelle. "Don't get drawn into one of those clunky all-or-nothing attitudes!"

WHO ARE YOU?

It's a good idea at the start to take your somatotype, or body type, into consideration because "working with your body is easier than working against it," says Michelle. Everyone has their own fat-to-muscle ratio and that means everyone's body has its own requirements for nutrition and training.

- **Ectomorphs** have narrower shoulders and hips in respect to their height, with relatively smaller muscles in respect to bone length. Their naturally fast metabolism can make it more challenging for these people to gain muscle mass. They can often tolerate slightly more carbs and lower amounts of fats.

- **Mesomorphs** have a medium bone structure, with shoulders wider than the hips. They have an efficient metabolism and a developed, athletic musculature. Their best diet is mixed, with a variety of fats, complex carbs, and proteins. They typically perform and feel best with a balance of all macronutrients.

- **Endomorphs** have stockier bone structures, with a larger midsection and hips, and they carry more fat throughout their bodies. They exhibit naturally slow metabolisms, which can be because of chronic conditions or as the result of a sedentary lifestyle. They typically have a lower carbohydrate tolerance and thus often benefit from a smaller intake of carbs and a higher intake of protein and fat.

Any body type needing to lose a significant percentage of body fat— or that has significant "stubborn fat" areas—will do best with a reduction of carbohydrates and fat, which can be figured into your macro-based nutrition plan.

Once you've used your nutrition plan—along with lifestyle modifications and physical training—to reach and maintain your desired body composition (weight, muscle build, muscle tone, etc.), you'll see that your body type has adapted to your "new normal." No one's body is static. Our appetites and our metabolisms adjust to energy intake and to physical output, and by the time you find yourself looking forward to your workout rather than seeing it as a chore, you might also be seeing some changes in your somatotype. In fact, someone predominately ectomorphic or endomorphic can over time present more mesomorphic traits.

WORKING WITH MACROS

We're as a culture woefully undereducated about the foods we eat. But it's important to understand the role of every macronutrient in your diet: They all serve different purposes and support your health and vitality in different ways. Consuming enough protein ensures you're either gaining or maintaining the maximum amount of metabolic-enhancing muscle mass. Consuming enough carbohydrates ensures you have enough muscle glycogen for energy to fuel effective workouts. (Always eat complex carbohydrates—preferably from foods high in fiber content—and avoid simple sugars.) Eat protein from many different sources in small portions throughout the day. A quality whey protein supplement is highly recommended because of its high biological value and generous supply of the branched-chain amino acids (BCAA) needed for energy.

These categories aren't as discrete as you might first assume. Most foods have a combination of macronutrients. For example, salmon is a protein that contains fat; dairy is a protein that contains carbs; and so on. While a general understanding of macronutrients is helpful, when you do start calculating your intake, you'll want to use an app (Michelle and Joan recommend My Macros+) that takes all of a given food's components into account. Fundamentally, though, here's what you consume every day:

- **Carbohydrates.** You'll find carbs in bread, fruit, vegetables, rice, pasta, potatoes, and legumes. Every gram of carb contains four calories. They're an important source of nutrients and fiber, and they're absolutely essential if you're going to exercise regularly. Carbs are your preferred source of quick energy and excess carbs can be stored in your muscles for fuel.

- **Protein.** You get protein from meat, chicken, fish, eggs, dairy, whey, and tofu. Every gram of protein contains four calories. So why do we need so much of it? It's because protein delivers a whole lot from those calories: It builds and maintains your immune system, it manufactures hormones, and it repairs body tissues. Your body will use 25% of the calories that are in protein to digest that same protein. It's your builder macro that protects your bones, your DNA, and your muscle mass. And, finally, you feel fuller after consuming protein, so you're a lot less likely to overeat.

- **Fat.** Many diets are intensely low fat and this can cause problems: You need fat in order to survive! You get it from oils, butter, nuts and nut butter, and avocados. Every gram of fat contains nine calories. Fat will help your body absorb vitamins (A, D, E, and K), produce and regulate hormones, and support cell growth. It's a source of long-term energy that can be used immediately as fuel (with the caveat that if it's not used, it will be stored as body fat!).

In addition to these macronutrients, your body requires micronutrients—vitamins and minerals—to support optimum health and vitality. It's always best if you can derive all your micronutrients from your diet (more on supplements later)—and that's easy: Just eat foods that include all the colors of the rainbow and you won't go wrong!

As with anything new, learning about and calculating your macros as well as learning to use your macros app will take time and attention at first. But you'll find it gets easier and easier the more you do it. Once you calculate your baseline macros, populate your food list, and have a few consistent days of planning your meals, you'll become more proficient and more efficient. The app will get easier and easier to use, and the progress you'll see will more than make up for the growing pains of learning a new skill.

LOOK AT THE SCIENCE

Macronutrient-based nutrition is rooted in science and much of what we've learned over the last few decades concerns protein.

Protein is essential for nurturing muscles, so this approach is entirely complementary to what you're doing in the gym. The ideal way of supporting muscle tissue is to consume protein every three hours. Of course, the amount of protein you consume varies, but there should be some in every one of the five meals you're enjoying every day.

"There's a lot of research out there focused on dosing protein for muscle development," says Michelle. "We're just following the science and we're always trying to optimize. Building muscle tissue is difficult, so we optimize nutrition to facilitate it. That means eating complete meals but never skimping on the protein.

"Think of it this way: Your food is really just a bowl of chemicals. Macro, micro, fiber. When you smell it, you're experiencing a cascade of bio receptors and responses—a cascade of hormones. What kind of cascade you experience can be affected by the combinations of food you're eating," she says.

Of course, it's not just protein that's affected by how you put your meal together. Your body's insulin needs are regulated by your blood glucose levels. Your glycemic load—the amount of carbs in a portion of food combined with the speed at which it raises blood glucose levels—needs to be monitored. "Carrots have a high glycemic index," says Michelle, "but also lots of fiber. You won't binge-eat on it. It won't cause a big disruption. It's things that are easy to overeat, like honey, that you need to keep an eye on."

So why not just juice and get all that goodness in a glass? "That's a problem," says Michelle. "You've taken foods in whole food form and you just removed the fiber. That's just not healthy. It's not going to keep your blood sugar level stable and it's not giving you your protein every three hours. So that's problematic. Plus, juice isn't filling."

This is all about your budget. You have *x* number of grams of protein, *x* number of grams of carbohydrates, *x* number of grams of fat. How do you want to spend them?

"Ask yourself: 'If I have that, will I be successful today?'" says Michelle. "'Is it satiating? If it isn't, then I'll eat more. I'll be creating cravings.' This is why we encourage you to educate yourself. How much do you like it? How much can you have?"

Designing your meal plan with your preferences in mind makes it more appealing, and if your meal plan doesn't feel restrictive, then what you have is a successful meal plan. "It has been such a huge hit for so many women," says Michelle. Some women have an initial resistance to weighing out the food, but "the chances of finding a recipe that's already perfect are slim," says Michelle. "Instead, get used to grams because they're the holy grail of the wide world of making the recipes work for you."

Using the My Macros+ app "just makes it easier," says Michelle. "The idea is you don't have to do much math. Just play with the dials and the app spits out the numbers. And a good kitchen scale will convert everything you need quickly and simply."

"You're not a victim to your diet," she adds. "Most people are undereating on protein and overeating on fat. We increase the protein and adjust the carbs and the fat. You can lose weight just by doing that. You can't argue with the results of thousands of clients."

How do you calculate and adjust your macros? Michelle's book *Macros Mastery* goes into that and many other aspects of macro-based eating and nutrition and offers all the information you need, including food lists and recipes crafted by this master chef, to truly "master" using macros. In the meantime, though, we can offer you ways of getting started right now.

GETTING STARTED

This is where you'll figure out your macro plan. You can do it alone or with the guidance of a trainer or nutritionist. No matter whether you do it on your own or with an expert or a group, here's what you need to do to get started.

First, you'll want to download a food-tracking app. Next, track everything you eat for two weeks. This doesn't just mean "two slices of bread, peanut butter, jelly." You need to look at how much of each food you're consuming and find information about the nutritional breakdown of your specific foods. You can use the My Macros+ app or a trusted online source to get the macro data you need to fill in your list.

Now you have your two weeks' data. What are your average daily calories? Wait—don't change them yet because you're first going to balance them among your macros!

In *Macro Mastery*, Michelle provides the following steps for creating and calculating your macros:

- Calculate your total protein intake by multiplying your ideal body weight by a factor of anywhere from 1 to 1.4. This will give you the total amount of daily protein you should be consuming in grams.

- Calculate your total dietary fat intake by taking your ideal body weight and multiplying it by a factor of anywhere from 0.3 to 0.5. This will give you the total amount of fat you should be consuming in grams.

- Carbs will make up the rest.

- Divide these macros into five meals.

- On training days, have more carbs before and after training, with a focus on starch, particularly starch that's easy to digest. Then taper your carbs throughout the remainder of the day. Your body naturally has better insulin sensitivity (that is, it can partition starch better) in the first part of the day. Spreading starch evenly throughout the day, with slightly more in the first part of the day and then tapering off toward the end of the day, is always a safe bet when starting on a fat loss journey.

- Split your protein evenly throughout the day. You can opt for slightly less protein in your pre- and postworkout meals if carbs are substantially high. This will allow for better digestion of carbs in those meals and more satiety from higher protein in later meals when carbs are lower. Ditto for fat. Spread it evenly through each meal, but you can bring it down slightly in the pre- and postworkout meals for the same reason as protein.

- Learning how to create balanced, micronutrient-rich meals is another key to longevity. For this reason, we encourage reserving a portion of the total carbohydrate contribution in a given meal for micronutrient-rich fibrous carbs, like vegetables. Of course, pre- and postworkout carbs should be predominately easy-to-digest starch, but in other meals, shift more focus to vegetables.

- For nontraining days, you want to consume about 150 to 250 fewer calories. This deficit should come from reducing the amount of carbohydrates you consume and you might also want to increase your fat macros slightly. At The Wonder Women, we take into account things like a client's waist circumference (a waist above 35 inches indicates poor insulin sensitivity), the intensity of the client's training sessions, her body type (an endomorph body type tends to lose body fat better with a lower-carb approach), and how much fat loss we're aiming for overall (the bigger the fat loss goal, the less likely a high-carb approach will work well). We also look at things like adherence, satiety, and palatability. If we can bring fat up a little bit on the lower-carb days and still achieve fat loss, this will likely allow for more variety and satisfaction from food choices because it opens up more protein sources and more condiment or fat choices.

- Each meal will be consumed two and a half to three hours apart. You'll want to monitor your progress by tracking metrics daily (weight as well as waist, hip, and thigh measurements) and taking weekly progress pics. Then you'll adjust your macro distribution based on changes in metrics and physique. Generally, small reductions in carb and fat macros will be prioritized for continued progress, and protein usually remains the same. The exception is when you need to reduce calories and the carbs and/or fat are already quite low. In this case, you'll need to reduce protein. Try to avoid going below 1 gram per 1 pound of ideal body weight for protein and certainly not less than 0.7 grams per 1 pound.

MICHELLE'S CASE STUDY

Cindy weighs 175 pounds, she's 5-foot-6, and her metrics are: waist 33 inches, hips 41 inches, and right thigh 25 inches.

Cindy has an endomorph body type. Her ideal body weight is 140 pounds. She tracked her food for two weeks and figured out she was consuming about 1,700 calories a day on average. Her protein consumption was decent at 150 grams per day.

- **Protein.** She decides to set her protein at 1.3 times her ideal body weight, or 180 grams. There are 4 calories per gram in protein, so this amounts to 720 calories (180 x 4 = 720).

- **Fat.** 140 x 0.4 = 56 grams. We'll round this to 55 grams for simplicity's sake. There are 9 calories per gram in fat, so this amounts to 495 calories (55 x 9 = 495).

- **Carbs.** 1700 – 720 – 495 = 485 calories left for carbs. There are 4 calories in every gram of carbohydrate, so this amounts to 121 grams of carbs a day, which we'll round to 120 for simplicity.

To summarize, macros for a training day will be: 180 grams of protein, 120 grams of carbs, and 55 grams of fat, or 1,695 calories.

If you divide this into five meals per the instructions above, it should give you something like this: Let's say Cindy will be doing four low-carb days per week because she knows she's an endomorph and will do better with lower carbs. That means she won't have as big of a drop in calories between her training and nontraining days right from the start.

	Pre-workout	Post-workout	Meal 3	Meal 4	Meal 5
Protein 180g	30g	30g	40g	40g	40g
Carbs 120g	30g 5g from fruit & veg is okay	30g 5g from fruit & veg is okay	25g 12.5g from starch is okay	25g 12.5g from starch is okay	10g
Fat 55g	8g	8g	13g	13g	13g

Therefore, we can reduce by just 135 calories and her nontraining day macros could look like this: 180 calories of protein, 75 grams of carbs, and 60 grams of fat, or 1,560 calories.

Cindy will continue to take and log her metrics each morning before eating and drinking to monitor her progress. Metrics include her weight as well as her waist, hip, and right thigh measurements. She'll adjust her macros based on how her metrics are moving and in what direction.

	Meal 1	Meal 2	Meal 3	Meal 4	Meal 5
Protein 180g	36g	36g	36g	36g	36g
Carbs 75g	20g 20g from starch is okay	15g 7.5g from starch is okay	15g 7.5g from starch is okay	15g 7.5g from starch is okay	10g
Fat 60g	12g	12g	12g	12g	12g

She can always make small calculated adjustments to her macros and calories for the day. Generally, protein will remain untouched, while carbs and fats will be adjusted first.

As you become more accustomed to planning and adjusting your macros, it will become easier and easier for you to do. And the best part is that it just works.

As one The Wonder Women participant says: "The science that Michelle applied to my macros and training evidenced itself each week, as I lost around 0.8 to 1 pound every Saturday morning. Every week, I took my 'celebration pictures.' It was mind-blowing to see the changes over time! This isn't a fad diet. Not low carb. Not low fat. Not keto. Not intermittent fasting. I'd tried all those things—and they didn't work. It was freedom with choosing enjoyable foods, preplanning them the night before, lovingly dosing my body throughout the day with six meals, savoring each bite, and enjoying the nutrients I was supplying to my muscles that had been working so hard throughout the week."

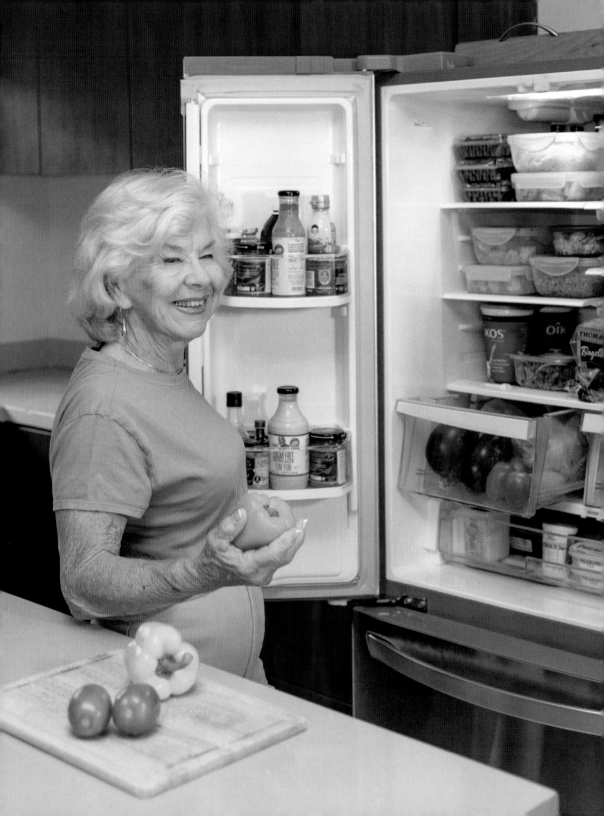

"We encourage our clients to learn how to use an app like My Macros+ to plan out meals that suit their own personal tastes while sticking to a macro budget for each meal," Michelle says. One of The Wonder Women participants adds: "The results have been outstanding. My body handles this kind of plan really well, and psychologically, I never feel restricted. Quite the opposite: I feel liberated from doubt, fear, and food anxiety because everything is planned and accounted for and there are no surprises—whether on the scale or with my health and vitality."

PLANNING YOUR MEALS TO FIT INTO YOUR SCHEDULE

A lot of women will look at this way of planning and organizing their meals and think, "Not with my family I won't!" Anyone who's raised children is familiar with the tyranny of the plate, wherein broccoli can never touch potatoes and any deviation from expected norms results in a fit of howling!

But it's easier to make this a part of your family routine than you might think. "So let's say your family wants spaghetti," says Michelle. "You just make the ground beef on the side. They'll have whatever they have, but you'll measure your food out." You end up sharing the same meal— the only difference being your family serves itself from the bowls on the table and you'll have premeasured your plate out. You'll use the same ingredients but with different amounts and possibly cooked differently.

As it turns out, some families are open to the idea of macro-based meals. "There are more and more instances now where the couple is following macros," says Michelle. "If you're in an adult household, it's fine to do different meals. Think about it this way: When we go out to a restaurant, the whole family doesn't order the same thing, right? You can do the same thing at home and it automatically removes all the tension."

Joan agrees. "When I'm in Mexico with my daughter and son-in-law, we'll all be in the kitchen doing our meal prep and we'll all be putting different things in our little Tupperware containers. Why not? We're each different and have different goals for our health."

Can vegetarians follow a macro-based nutrition program? "Absolutely!" says Michelle. "You should prioritize whole foods. That's food as nature intended it. It means using olives instead of olive oil. No protein bars. And as a vegetarian, it might mean rethinking your ingredients and understanding protein powerhouses. For example, wheat has more protein than rice. Prioritize mushrooms or broccoli over tomatoes. Instead of using oil, choose nuts. You'll also want to make use of a quality protein powder supplement. But it's all doable."

There are some professions or work environments in which following the schedule might be more challenging than others. "I'm thinking of a busy nurse," says Michelle, "or a serious dogwalker. But those are easy adjustments to make. We can still work it out with protein shakes—they're not smelly or difficult to prepare. If you work in an office or anywhere with a kitchen area, just prepare your small meals in advance and reheat them at the office. If you don't have a fridge, there are insulated bags with separate pockets for cooling gel packs, Tupperware containers, even a space for vitamins. The meals can stay in there all day."

Another practical challenge is around traveling. "You just have to plan in advance," says Joan. "Figure out how many meals you have to make and prep them the day before you go. The only issue is around choosing foods that taste good without needing to be cooked. I always bring small containers of my favorite foods: pasta, ratatouille, a rice dish, broccoli and pork with soy sauce. It's all easy to eat—and super yummy!"

Preparing and consuming meals at home might involve less planning than you need with away-from-home meals, but you still want to be efficient. Michelle recommends organizing your refrigerator so you have easy access to your premeasured ingredients.

"Start with quality condiments you know the macros for," she says. "And keep your shelves organized. Have an uncooked vegetable and fruit drawer. Another drawer for fats. And a shelf for cooked protein— pork tenderloin, cooked chicken on the bone, salmon. It's easy to just cook up several proteins at once and store them for the next couple days." This is especially important given the emphasis on protein as necessary for building muscle.

"Have a dairy shelf," Michelle continues. "And then an upper drawer with prepared carbs, carrot soup, ratatouille, rice noodles, berry compote, all your starches."

There's a reason for this level of organization. Because you'll often be preparing more than one meal at a time, the last thing you need is to suddenly realize you don't have a key ingredient. "It makes for a lot of ease in seeing when you need more," says Michelle.

Food preparation doesn't have to take long. "It's super efficient to do a lot of food prep at once, get your oven and two pots going, because then you're topping off your food and being prepared all the time," says Michelle. But you don't have to wait until you have two hours blocked off in your schedule. "I call it slipping it in the cracks," she says. "You can do it a little at a time. If you have 10 minutes between a call and a class, you can do a little food prep. Slipping it in the cracks of your schedule. I like to have food fresh, so I'm just always doing a little at a time."

And if you do find you're missing that "key" ingredient, it doesn't have to be a problem. "You can usually substitute something else when necessary if you can't go to the grocery store," says Michelle. "Or maybe you're in a rush. Rice noodles take three minutes to cook, so you can use them instead of rice. They're just as yummy and they're ready in no time."

She emphasizes that getting to know your ingredients, general cooking times, and being organized will all keep you from getting thrown off course. This includes shopping. "Make sure you and everyone in your household uses the same terminology," she says. "Speaking the same language helps when you send someone to the store."

Meal planning is associated with increased food variety—a key component of a healthy diet that increases the likelihood of meeting nutrient needs and making healthy eating a lot less dull. Perhaps even more importantly, cooking at home also gives you control and choice over ingredients.

For busy people, it's a matter of getting organized—and having fallback plans. "There are companies that do macro-based food. That's another option," says Michelle. But what it comes down to mostly is developing a new way of thinking about meals and meal preparation and organizing your prep time around that. "Remember you're switching a lot of ingredients in and out," says Michelle. "One day, you might have beef, rice noodles, and broccoli. You can change out the beef for salmon or switch to rice for your carbs. These are small, easy swaps that give you flexibility and different flavors. They keep things interesting. Swap in any fresh items you have—they're the best."

EQUIPMENT

Meal preparation will be stress-free, efficient, simple, and even fun as long as you have the right tools. Michelle recommends the following:

- air fryer
- baking dish
- baking sheet
- cooling rack
- cutting board
- food scale
- grater
- kitchen timer
- large chef's knife
- leak-proof food containers

- measuring cups and spoons
- meat thermometer
- mini food processor
- nonstick skillets
- nonstick spatula
- pots
- silicone muffin mold
- strainers
- tongs
- wooden spoons

As you become more familiar with cooking and food preparation around macros, you'll no doubt find some utensils and equipment will become your favorites.

Finally, it's ultimately about what you bring to the experience that will make all the difference. "We craft macros for each meal to make sure all the bars line up, but you're the one putting them together—and, seriously, how clever are you for getting things in line?" What you'll see is a development of pride in the way you're making the program work and in the quality of food that you're putting together. "That's worth sharing!" says Michelle. "Show your pride. Instagram it! Share screenshots and photos and recipes. Put some hashtags on so others can be inspired by what you're doing."

You might have begun this journey with uninteresting food on your plate, but as your repertoire and your enthusiasm build, you'll be creating amazing meals. Give yourself some credit for that!

WHAT ABOUT SUPPLEMENTS?

If you're following a balanced macro-based diet, you probably won't need much in the way of supplements. So if you're wondering about what "extras" your body needs, look first to your food.

Older women are generally not eating a lot of food that's high in quality protein, which can result in many of them requiring supplements. They also tend to not eat the full spectrum of "rainbow" vegetables and use oils rather than whole food fats. There's nothing wrong with taking a quality multivitamin, says Michelle, but beware: "The vitamin industry is unregulated, so be cautious. Make sure the company you buy from does third-party testing and observe the clinical dosage of supplements to get the dosage you want. Thorne is an example of a company that works in the medical field as well as supplements, so they'll deliver an effective dosage. Do your homework."

There are some supplements that Michelle feels might be useful at different points on your journey or at different times of the day:

- A fish oil supplement (omega-3 fatty acid) can be helpful.

- Evening primrose, also rich in the omega chain fatty acids, has anti-inflammatory and antioxidant properties.

- For the nighttime, she recommends taking calcium/magnesium, which helps you feel calm, promotes better sleep, and helps your bowels stay healthy.

- Speaking of which, a fiber supplement like Benefiber and Metamucil helps with motility for women.

- When you're doing serious weight training (and she means *serious*, like when Joan is thrusting 200 pounds!), 5 grams of creatine can help sustain high-intensity workouts.

- For fat loss, green tea extract helps improve fatty acid metabolism. Take 1000 to 2000 milligrams in the early part of the day.

- Caffeine also helps improve fatty acid metabolism. Use 2 to 9 grams per kilogram of weight. Start with the lowest amount and see how it goes.

"I've tried different supplements," says Joan. "I've taken glucosamine chondroitin for arthritis. Vitamin C. B-50 sometimes. Actually, I do supplements mainly for arthritis: Turmeric and cumin are good for it, and cinnamon's an excellent anti-inflammatory. You can slow it down, but you can't stop it entirely unfortunately."

There are supplements that are especially important when you're changing your physique. "When you're building muscle, you tear your muscles and then they grow when you're sleeping," says Joan. "So I take a BCAA [branched-chain amino acid] supplement that helps with muscle growth."

Other supplements Joan uses include collagen peptides. "My skin looks better when I'm taking that regularly," she says. "You can't stop the wrinkles though—unfortunately! But as I like to say, I earned every one of them!"

In addition to the fiber Michelle recommends, Joan adds items to keep her gut healthy. "I drink Smooth Move tea," she says. "And proactive greens. A lot of us have that problem with the gut. Doctors don't know a lot about nutrition. It's not their fault. They're taught how to fix things. But why let something get bad if you can prevent it from happening in the first place? That's been a major shift in my thinking personally. Preventative medicine should be practiced more and keep the rest for when something goes wrong. Stop things happening first!"

By and large, though, both women agree that keeping supplements to a minimum and getting your micronutrients through your food is the best course of action. "Try to balance out your meals so you don't need the supplements! The macros provide that balance," says Joan. "I know that nursing homes have removed a lot of protein from their menus and that's a problem for most people because then they eat too many carbs and too much sugar."

While too much processed sugar isn't the only culprit, it's right up there. "You could stop people from getting a sweet tooth if you start from babyhood," argues Joan. "It's an acquired taste. Years ago, rich people had rotten teeth because they could afford sugar and the poor weren't allowed sugar and they were often in better shape! It's all over the place—in gravies and sauces. Once you start really looking, you'll find sugar everywhere. We've done this to ourselves over the centuries. That's a lot of repetitive bad habits! But now we're trying to enlighten people. You have to unravel centuries of habits and we're trying to do it in years. It's a mammoth task." But she has a lot of hope: "Change a few million people and they can change a few million and then it might change going forward."

The "supplements" Joan really likes to talk about are all for flavor. "I use a little salt," she says. "Mostly in the cooking water. Salt's so addictive, I try to stay away from it. I do love those steak seasoning/chicken seasoning blends. And herbes de Provence—there's nothing like a ratatouille with herbes de Provence. I do that one by memory now, I make it so often! I also love pesto and use it in a lot of things."

HOW TO HANDLE DISRUPTIONS

Of course, not every day is going to go according to plan. All sorts of disruptions can get between you and your lifestyle choices. It's going to happen—guaranteed.

But while disruptions are guaranteed to happen, they don't have to throw you off.

One common disruption to your plan is illness. Whether it's a winter cold or something more severe, you're not going to feel like measuring food or preplanning meals. "If you're battling illness, your priority is to get better," says Michelle. "Anything else is secondary to that. So follow the course of action recommended by your doctor."

When you're ill, you'll often lose your appetite, so Michelle recommends what she calls the "BRAT diet": broth, white rice, applesauce, and toast—simple to digest and high in carbohydrates. "Don't get too stressed about cooking protein while you're sick," says Michelle. "Keep hydrated and rest."

While you'll probably be eating less when you're ill, if you're recovering from an injury, you'll want to be eating more food to support your body's healing process. This is especially true after surgery of any kind. "Focus on getting better," says Michelle. "You might have dropped off calories to keep progressing—say you're consuming 1,200—bring that back up to 2,000. You can still have pride in your food and your nutrition. Don't undereat or go off plan—you don't need to do that—but just allow your body to heal. And our plan is so balanced, it really gives you a great blueprint for taking care of yourself."

Then there's the disruption we all encounter and possibly dread the most: the psychological disruption. For some reason, you've gone off plan. You've had wine with dinner. You've given in to that alluring dessert. And now the guilt is flooding in.

First of all, use that newly developed self-awareness you've been practicing to help you put the brakes on and coach yourself through the experience, Michelle suggests. There are simple strategies that work. "Take a sip of sparkling water between every sip of wine," she says.

"Use a smaller plate at the buffet and only go up once." You can also read the menu and plan your meal beforehand so you don't give in to the momentary pressure of a beautiful dessert cart.

The essential question to defer to is this: What do I want out of this experience? Once you've answered that question, all the other decisions fall into line behind it. "You can still have a social life. You can still enjoy yourself without messing up your week," says Michelle.

Of course, plans do go awry—even the best ones—and sometimes you will, in fact, mess up. Michelle's advice: Get right back on the horse. "Have some perspective," she says. "You have 35 meals in a week. If you get one or even two wrong, it's not going to undo all the others." The goal here is to avoid anxiety and binary thinking about your process. "Think of what you'd say to a child who made a mistake," says Michelle. "You'd deal with them with compassion, right? So give yourself that same compassion. You can self-coach—you know the things to say. And then this will help you build a better strategy."

You can take slips as evidence that you need some more strategies. "Just have perspective," says Michelle. "Pick up where you left off. Stick to the plan and it will come right naturally."

"It happens to everyone," says Joan. "The key is to not let your feelings overwhelm you. You can go down a rabbit hole of guilt. Don't do that."

NUTRITION & DISEASE

"People just aren't educated on the elements of food," says Joan. "I'm still learning about food and what you can and can't put together. You don't need a lot of spices—just three or four—to change up the taste.

You don't need to fry anything. Use an air fryer—that heat's just flying around and it's done in no time flat with no grease. These are really simple things, but in decades of dieting, I never learned about them."

And they relate to the way our bodies handle injuries, illness, and diseases. "Most doctors are general practitioners and so they don't specialize," Joan says. "They can't possibly know everything. So when you go to your doctor and they don't know these things—well, it's not their fault. They're taught to cure and to heal, not to keep the body from doing those things in the first place."

She speaks from experience. "I was on blood pressure medication for 15 years," Joan says. "I saw what my dad went through—he was on so many medications and I thought 'That can't be good.' I don't want any dependency on drugs, but what else was I going to do? I had bad acid reflux, my kidneys had already failed, my doctor put me on a maintenance dosage for bad cholesterol."

And then she began her transformation program with her daughter. "I really was in bad shape," she admits. "My waist was 39 inches— anything over 36 is considered obese—and Michelle told me, 'You have to get that waistline down for your health.' I listened to her because I didn't want to end up in a nursing home like my mother did. And you know what? Within the first year, I lost weight, I lost inches, and I was completely off my blood pressure medication. My BP was normal."

Giving your body a level of fitness at which it is more equipped to fight off illness and recover from injury is the best gift you can give yourself. It's one that will keep rewarding you for years.

The real wonder drug isn't your nutrition plan by itself—it's the combination of macro nutrition and healthy exercise. You can lower your blood pressure, lower your cholesterol, decrease arthritis pain, reduce your risk of injury from falls, decrease inflammation, and—best of all—feel great. "My mother is healthier now than she was 20 years ago," says Michelle.

Isn't that something you'd like for yourself?

MINDFUL EATING

It's no surprise to learn that many of us don't practice mindful eating. Western culture tends to discourage doing anything mindfully, least of all eating.

But practicing it is core to the success of your nutrition program.

Michelle was for many years a yoga instructor and competition participant before she turned to bodybuilding and she integrates that background with her current practices and those she teaches to others, including her mother. "My own long journey with yoga made me more mindful." And while she found that yoga wasn't as helpful in the areas of longevity and robust vitality and health, she did bring the concept of mindfulness with her. "It's actually an idea I developed for myself back when I was a binge eater," she explains. "And then later, when I was working in restaurants, I was seeing how people interact around food. And I realized there was a big breakdown around social eating especially."

Mindfulness in eating, like mindfulness in general, starts with gratitude—and gratitude alone can go a long way in making you feel better. It's been linked to some amazing outcomes, such as strengthening your immune system, improving sleep patterns, feeling optimistic, being more helpful and generous to others, and feeling less lonely and isolated. What's not to like?

"It's not unlike saying grace," says Michelle. "You start your meal with gratitude for what you're about to eat, the hands that grew and prepared it, the taste, everything." In these first moments, think about what food means to you: food as nourishment, food as medicine, food as creating muscle for you.

"You have to slow down," says Joan. "People eat without even tasting their food. I want to taste every morsel! You can only do all that when you slow down."

Slowing down involves taking your meals seriously—as events. "Even if you're eating alone, it's still a ritual," says Michelle. "Make a dinner setting for yourself. Use a nice glass, nice plates. Be present to the food you're preparing. Take some pride in plating it."

Once you're eating, pay attention. Take a bite of food and immediately put your fork down. Chew the food. Savor it. Think about it. Next, take a sip of water. Put down the glass, pause, and now pick up your fork for your next bite. If you're with someone, maintain eye contact and let the conversation become part of your ritual.

"You have to put your silverware down between every bite," says Joan. "That's a huge part of this mindfulness. And I think it's new to most people. Not to Europeans. They always eat that way. But North

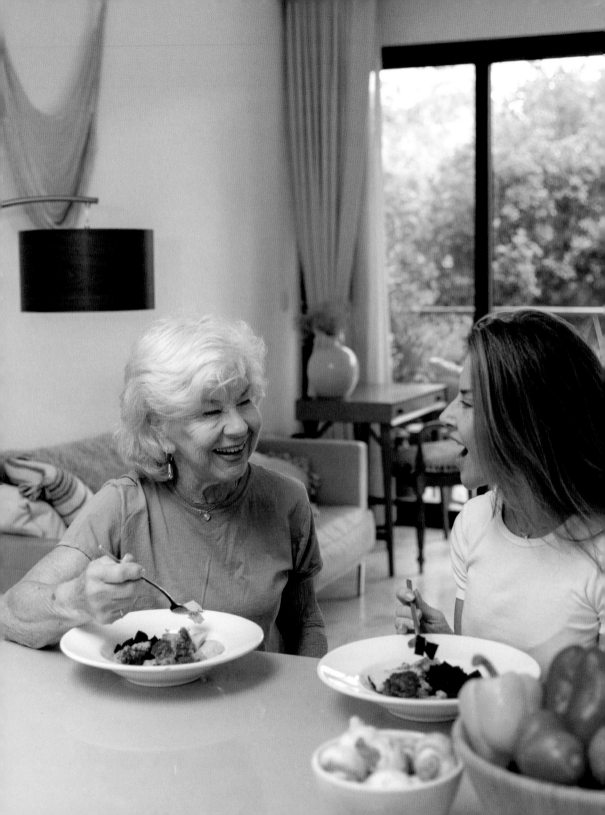

Americans, not so much. Imagine a video camera following you and recording you while you're eating. Imagine that! You'd be shocked at what you saw. We've lost all our manners."

There are so many things to notice when you eat. The texture of the food. Its taste. How it pairs with other things on your plate. People tasting wine and whiskey are attuned to identifying precisely when and where the flavors hit their tongues, their mouths. They take the time to identify every second of the experience.

What if we all ate our meals with the same care and consideration sommeliers take at wine tastings? "I'm a person who'd have my hot food hot and get it in fast," says Joan. "You don't taste it that way. Sit, have a conversation, make eye contact, have a sip of water and a forkful of food, make sure you chew properly, put the fork down. Do it again. You want to taste the food. I love the taste of food!"

Even your posture while eating makes a difference. "You want to elongate your spine," says Michelle. "That allows for better systems communication throughout your body. Your breath work is always important, so don't neglect it when you're eating. Research shows how quickly deep breathing calms your body and your mind."

Mindfulness will help not just with how you eat but also with how much you eat. Eating too quickly bypasses satiety cues your body is giving you—and you nearly always eat too much when you eat too fast.

"We teach all this," says Michelle. "Noticing yourself. Chewing, putting food on your fork, slowing down. Notice if you're not participating in the conversation. Eating mindfully creates self-awareness—and creates richness in a family setting or anytime you're eating food with others."

Mindful eating can also lead to new discoveries because you're truly tasting and thinking about what you're putting in your body. "I'm willing to try dishes I'd never had before," says Joan. "Grilled octopus? I'd never have put that in my mouth before. Calamari, the same. Not something you had normally. I love tapas. They allow you to try lots of things. Same with sushi. I even ate eel! Really? In the old days, I would've run a mile rather than eat eel. This blows my mind: I tried something so foreign and liked it! It's a real life lesson, isn't it?"

Being more strategic and mindful around food will support the rest of your life: your fitness goals, your social interactions, even your intimacy. Michelle remembers a participant who went out to dinner on a date night with her husband—and went off plan. "She was consumed with anxiety, shame, and guilt. What a difference from what that date night might have looked like—a night of romance at a fabulous restaurant." Staying on track with your goals is supported by being mindful, especially in unusual situations. "Instead, really enjoy the atmosphere, the company," says Michelle. "My husband and I have dinners out that last for two or three hours—and we don't drink alcohol. We tell the waiters to bring our food out slowly. We're completely present to the moment and to each other."

Being completely present to the moment drives a wedge into any triggered behavior around food consumption. It allows for pure enjoyment of the whole experience around an event—enjoying the anticipation, enjoying the dinner in the moment, enjoying later reflecting on the experience. This is what will last. It has to happen in your head—through your identity shift into the person you want to become and through mindfulness.

"We might start transforming from the outside, but the really amazing work is done on the inside," says Joan. "It's self-talk. Maybe you used to call yourself lazy and stupid, but you have to stop talking like that. This is my sixth year. It's taken a long time to change that kind of talking to myself. It was almost like a reflex, saying that. I don't really think I'm stupid, but I tended to say I was. But I'm not! I'm the only person who can give myself a healthy life. Whatever outcome you have is of your own making."

MOTIVATION

"Food is your medicine," says Michelle. "If you could use only one tool, choose food, not exercise. I want people to own their nutrition. Macros give you so much freedom to be so creative and answer your own needs, and when you use the app, it crunches the numbers for you—so it's easy. My clients serve meals I've created to others and none of it tastes like health food, which is a big asset, especially for moms!"

The best motivation is in the outcome. "Owning your nutrition, you'll get results that will serve you as motivation," says Michelle.

Her focus around motivation is in a person's ability to touch base with the passion they feel for their *why*. *Why* are you reading this book? *Why* did you pick up the Train with Joan app? *Why* are you willing to make an entire lifestyle change? If you can't answer the *why*, your motivation is sure to flag in the long run.

Know your *why*. Flesh it out. There are a lot of questions that feed into it: what you hope to achieve; what your future looks like. "It can't be someone else's," says Michelle. "For my mom, the *why* was wanting to get off medication—she had such a fear of taking more and more pills after seeing how her own mother ended up. Another gal wanted to be a great role model for her son and have the energy to keep up with him. Whatever yours is, keep coming back to it."

Once Joan had her *why*—better health naturally without medication—she and her coach determined a strategy that would get her there and set up some benchmark goals. She wanted to get her waist below 35 inches and to stop taking medications, so they broke those goals up into monthly and even weekly steps. "Every day when I get up, I have a checklist of things to do," says Joan.

"You become process-oriented every day to develop habits you need for the bigger *why*," says Michelle.

Too many people confuse motivation with discipline.

"Discipline is what you rely on when your motivation wanes," says Michelle. "Habits and passion are what you rely on to keep that motivation constant. Habit will get you an okay job, but add passion and you're unbeatable. Layer the passion on the habit and touch base with your *why* on a daily basis."

She's a prime example herself. "I love what I'm doing. I'm exactly where I want to be. The rewards are endless. I make everything I have to do fun every day so everything's infused with joy." How does she do that? "I do it with an internal narrative. Your internal dialogue can only be effective when your goal is aligned with your identity."

In other words, the *why*. The *why* of what you're doing and what you want as an outcome. The shift from "who you are now" to "who you can become."

Occasionally in life, you'll come across someone you admire—a mentor perhaps—someone who opens your mind and heart to things you might never before have considered, perhaps even didn't know existed. Something completely outside the scope of your own experience. It could be a career choice. It could be moving somewhere new. Whatever it is, if it attracts you, then there's a shift in perspective.

Michelle refers to it as a shift in identity. "You decide you're going to be that person," she says. "You can think your career into existence. Or your health. You start using the power of visualization and identify yourself deeply with that vision. That's where authentic passion and motivation come from. It's not about faking it until you make it. It's about identifying with the person you're becoming. Thoughts create reality. Once you start seeing the world through that lens, then challenges become springboards to growth."

She has some suggestions for keeping your motivation high:

- Flesh out your goal—find your *why* and believe in it.

- Make the identity shift. If you think a hangover is normal, it's time to take a leap of faith into something you've forgotten: what it feels like to feel healthy. Look at someone with robust health and vitality—and trust it's right for you. It's okay to burn bridges along the way—this is a new you you're creating and becoming.

- Infuse the things you have to be excited about with passion and joy. If you can train your mind to always look for the joy, it's a fabulous experience. Stressful situations don't continue to faze you and you can lean on the joy to help you make good decisions.

Training your mind is your ticket out of a state of anxiety or stress. It's not unlike training your pets. As someone with two new puppies in the family, Michelle can attest to this. "It's tough doing the training right," she says. "You want to give in to them. But if you do the work, if you stick to the schedule, then in a couple months, you'll have these two young dogs who'll be an absolute bundle of joy."

The process of training your mind isn't so very different. "You need to teach yourself the skills you'll use to guide yourself, using science, humor, passion, encouragement," says Michelle. "If you feel resentful or victimized or restricted by following these strategies, then you haven't yet had that identity shift. You have this beautiful piece of machinery and you didn't know how to use it. It's a great remote control device, but you couldn't enjoy all the channels. Here's the user manual, here's the blueprint to get there step-by-step."

Your mindset is the real game changer. Because success leaves a path, surrounding yourself with people who are more successful than you will inspire you to keep going, even when what you're doing feels a little like you're acquiring a foreign language.

"My mother's an icon to so many other women because it's not all that inspiring to see a 30-year-old get into shape," says Michelle. "She's an icon because there are women out there in their 50s and 60s who think it's impossible to get in shape because of their age. Mom's in her 70s, she's successful, so she inspires others."

And in the worst-case scenario, on the mornings you get up and just feel discouraged or low on energy, you'll still have your routine to fall back on. "Even when I travel, I get up every morning and still go through my checklist," says Joan. "It keeps me aware of myself and who I am. I'm someone who's developed good habits. I'm someone who can succeed." Over time, you'll develop the kind of repertoire of tools that will enable you to make the best possible choice in any situation. You'll have that internal support.

"I always encourage journaling and meditation for grounding," says Michelle. "But I also ask clients to create a list I call your 'aha moments.' They're your moments of clarity, and if you pay attention, those moments will give you tricks and tips you can use in any situation. It's a treasure trove of inspiration you've consciously built for yourself."

There's another list she also encourages making—one that will shrink with time. "It's what didn't work," says Michelle. "Maybe you didn't set boundaries. Maybe you weren't prepared for something. Maybe you overate. You learn from it, but first, you've got to feel the pain of it. The first time you do it, it's a mistake. The second time is a choice. The third time is a habit—and now it's a problem. Problems like that are indicators that you've shifted your attention away from the identity you're creating."

So keep your *why* in mind. Keep your new identity—the person you're going to become—at the forefront of your thoughts. Remind yourself of it when you start your day and when you end it.

"Thinking macros are the key to transformation is like thinking having a budget is the key to getting rich," says Joan. "You're missing the point. You can have the best-laid plan with the best coach, but it won't mean much if you don't become the person who thrives on following the plan. Success is an inside job and it will always, always come down to you."

Lesley Christensen

I discovered Train with Joan on Instagram and I was immediately hooked. I was 57 and feeling my age and figured it was going to be all downhill from there. But I looked at Joan and thought, "If she can do it, I can do it." I was the person who had the most weight to lose in our group. Michelle created a program that's a real boon to people like me who didn't know where to turn. She really inspires faith in people, makes you believe you can do it. And Joan is a like an icon for all of us, an example of what can be done. To be able to say "I trained with Joan MacDonald" is so amazing. She inspires so many people!

I kept going thanks to my teammates. We talked a lot in the chat and we posted collages of our photos every week in our Facebook group. No one wanted to do that, but we all had to do it—and it got less scary every week. We got used to seeing each other in our bikinis and talking about making progress. That just snowballed, compounded over time. Seeing the successes of my teammates was huge.

Now I'm weight training 5 times a week, I do cardio 3 times a week, and I do 8,000 steps every day. That's sustainable for me. I used to constantly be thinking about my weight and it felt like such a burden knowing I had to do something about it. I don't carry that burden anymore. I know what to do to maintain what I have—and my sanity along with it! I don't have to worry about motivation anymore. I know my habits will carry me forward.

So much has changed. I'll give you two examples. A huge motivator for me to get started was terrible back pain. I couldn't ride my motorcycle for any length of time—it hurt too much—but now I can do a weekend ride and it's fine. The second example of change is my brother's recent wedding. I'm actually looking forward to seeing the photos! I've gone from hiding in the back of group photos to not giving it a second thought.

Michelle's program is extraordinary. She makes us believe we can do it. She doesn't sugarcoat, she doesn't say it will be easy, she doesn't dumb anything down. She allows us to be self-motivated and figure things out. Michelle and Joan inspire such confidence. They changed my life.

CHAPTER SIX:

INTEGRATING YOUR NEW LIFESTYLE

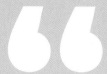

What I love about this lifestyle is I just keep feeling better about life. My sleep is better, my mood and energy are better, my appetite is much better, and I don't feel the walls closing in on me anymore.

Joan MacDonald

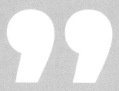

Everything we've been talking about—working out, following a macro-based nutrition plan, changing your mindset along with your lifestyle—comes together in one fundamental health consideration: your emotional well-being.

Did you know that depression is the fourth-leading cause of disability worldwide? There are myriad "kinds" of depression—from clinical depression that needs to be addressed in a professional setting to frequent attacks of the "blues." Combining exercise and sensible eating habits that support your body and general health will go a long way toward alleviating negative feelings.

The way to do it is to see your eating and exercise habits not as something you do but as part of your lifestyle. They're part of who you are at your most fundamental. They're the cornerstone on which everything else is built. Using these habits as a foundation on which to construct the rest of your life will ensure vitality and energy in everything you do. Combining the weight training necessary to build and keep strong muscles with everyday exercise and movement will alleviate depression and anxiety (which are, after all, two sides of the same coin) and can prevent their onset.

Food gives you energy—and you need energy to exercise. The emotional benefits of combining them are greater than the sum of their parts. When you exercise, you produce a "cocktail" of hormones that help you feel good. Endorphins are produced at a certain intensity of activity, but the mood-boosting effects of exercise are felt at a much lower level. "Getting healthy is about so much more than losing weight and looking good, although those are very nice things," says Joan. "Getting healthy impacts your entire attitude toward life, your alertness, and your optimism."

"One thing I learned through all this is that we make time for what we want to make time for," says one The Wonder Women participant. "Everyone has time to do what they want to do. It's a matter of choice." But it's true that for many of us, just starting a new challenging book— or even a TV series—can be a challenge; so how can we find the time to make space in our lives and schedules for something life-changing?

We give time and energy to what we care about. It's really that simple. Where we spend our time—our most precious commodity—says everything about who we are, what our priorities are, and the present and future we want for ourselves.

You usually do manage to fit in that book or TV program, right? You'll manage this too—and it will be more fulfilling than you ever imagined!

HOW FITNESS & NUTRITION WORK TOGETHER

Nutrition and exercise not only complement each other, but they also need each other. Even if you eat a perfectly balanced diet, you need to exercise to burn the calories. You also need to exercise to strengthen your muscles, heart, and lungs.

"Balance is dynamic," says Michelle. "It's not a static state of affairs. Rather, it's a constant adjustment to stimuli to maintain a certain state of homeostasis. It's also going to look very different between different people. What's balanced for me might not be maintainable for another woman and vice versa."

It seems cliché to say—but bears repeating—that working out can help improve your overall health and fitness level. There are a lot of studies out there showing how regular exercise can reduce the risk of developing chronic ailments, like heart disease, stroke, and diabetes. In addition, exercise lowers your stress and anxiety levels. "People reach for food or alcohol when they're feeling stressed," says Joan. "But even if they get a fix from that, it's only temporary. The effects of a good workout last longer, and if you keep doing it, they'll last a lifetime!"

Plus, starting a workout routine can be a great way to meet new people and make new friends. Working out with others can make the experience more enjoyable and motivating. "These days, I exercise like my life depends on it," says Joan. "And you know what? It does! I'll never give up fitness now. The rewards are endless!"

Keep that balance going: healthy eating, weights, cardio. Count your steps. Go to the gym. Drink lots of water. Have fun with life! "You don't have to believe what you've been told," says Joan. "You can change the story. It's only true if you make it true. Most people just want a quiet life and that's so defeating. You have to rock the boat or you're never going to get anywhere."

WHY THIS APPROACH WORKS

One of the strengths of a program like Joan follows, which works with lifestyle changes, is its emphasis on building muscle. Everything else flows from that: weight loss, toning, food choices, self-esteem. One of the most common misconceptions about women lifting weights is that it will make you bulky. It simply isn't true: A woman's body isn't naturally designed to build large amounts of muscle mass, so it's very unlikely that you'll bulk up from lifting weights. "Building muscle is a slow process. You can't see muscle growth a little at a time, although that's how it happen," Michelle says.

In fact, lifting heavier weights can help burn more calories and provide an amazing muscle definition that gives you the toned look everyone wants. Start with a challenging, manageable weight if you're new to lifting. Then you can gradually increase the amount of weight you're using and focus on your form.

Spacing your meals, using your food before it can translate into fat stores, and generally keeping your blood sugar level constant also contribute to building muscle—all of which can also improve your mood.

Finally, the community built and experienced by participants keeps everyone on track and feeling supported.

"We're not gifted with knowing how to have life with abundance," says Michelle. "It's absolutely a mindset. None of this is going to work if you don't integrate it with your mindset. Ask yourself the important questions: What's your purpose in life? What do you want to do in the world that brings meaning and value?"

Most people don't ask those questions or don't ask them in the context of overall health and vitality. "No wonder we're all out of alignment!" says Michelle. "Muscles aren't ours naturally—we've all seen how quickly we can get out of shape. We have to work to maintain muscle. You could survive by never eating anything but what you can get at McDonald's—but that's not living. My mom was on the verge of giving up gardening, which she loved, and now she's bursting with energy and joy. It's the structure that's important. Asking yourself the meaningful questions. That's very different from just going and picking up weights at the gym."

That structure isn't just about mindset though. It's also about following some very basic rules. You're not randomly eating less or heading out for a run from time to time. Your fitness and nutrition need to be structured. "It's really simple," says Michelle. "Do 10 to 12 sets of 4 exercises for each body part in 4 workouts per week. Be sure to hit the whole body at least once a week. There's great information for all this online. Check it out. And just make sure you get better over time."

What does that mean? "It's a system called 'progressive overload,'" she says. "Your body adapts, so you have to keep challenging it. The training stress has to keep increasing." You can increase that stress in a number of ways: adding weight, adding repetitions, shortening your rest periods, focusing on the perfect form, improving your range of motion. "It doesn't have to be complicated. Just hit your entire body with a selection of quality exercises," says Michelle.

"That training is creating stress on your body," she continues. "Your muscles go through a series of reactions if the stress is hard enough. Then your body rebuilds itself with better, stronger muscles."

Along with your mindset and your determination to grow into the person you want to be in the world, be very invested in being consistent. "Better to do something you can follow," says Michelle. "Three workouts a week is the minimum, four is better, and five is great for fast, visible results that will help you stay motivated. Any woman is going to see amazing results with five workouts a week."

And while many people are conditioned to see workouts as perhaps a necessary but not particularly joyful part of their transformations, they're not taking the release of endorphins that weight exercise provides into account. "New lifters don't always get it," says Michelle.

"Every day, I can't wait to get back to my routine. I love how I feel when I train. And exercise is the best antidote for depression and anxiety."

Another reason a program like this works is that it gives structure to your day. This can be helpful for anyone, but it's especially meaningful and even life-changing for those who have to deal with a level of chaos in their lives. Your workouts and your meals will require you to set a schedule and establish boundaries.

"Either way, you'll be in better shape," says Michelle. "But when everything's combined, it's synergistic. You'll make more progress, which will give you more positive feedback, which will help you make more progress, and so on." And it shows. "Some gals have been asked if they'd had plastic surgery—this progress shows in their faces, in better oxygenation, in better sleep. You get hormonal benefits, restructuring benefits, and faster and better results."

When you divide your food into five meals a day, you're creating muscle protein synthesis because you're consuming protein every three hours. The meals are balanced, meaning your blood sugar will remain relatively stable without highs and lows. "We want you hungry—but not so hungry you'll break your diet or becoming hyperglycemic and jittery," says Michelle. The practice also avoids anyone having a lot of calories in one sitting.

The workouts support that. "If muscle cells aren't being trained to exhaustion, there's no inclination for them to absorb glucose, so the fat cells get it instead. The more muscle you have, the more you train, the more you're able to handle a big-calorie meal."

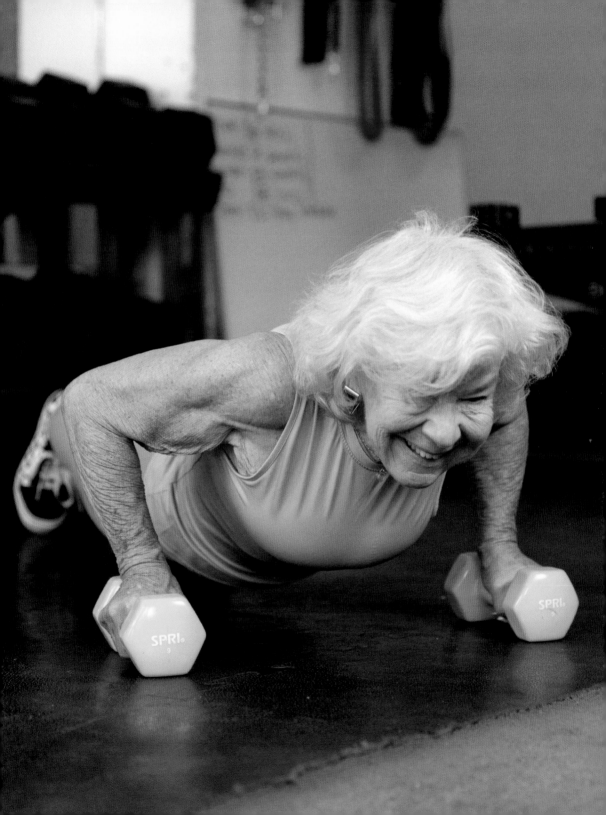

The timing of those meals makes a difference. Right after a training session, when your muscles are close to failure, there's a window of about 45 minutes when they're sensitive and can handle more calories. "When we do a leg session, right after the workout, we bike to the ice cream shop," says Michelle. "The exact right time is postworkout because the fat digests fast—it just evaporates. People eat salad after they train—that's exactly backward. You really can have your cake and your six-pack too."

She admits the choice isn't always obvious. "Sometimes, clients see me as a last chance," she says. "They're skeptical. But what they begin to see is what's on the other side: excitement, hope, optimism about what's next. Every weekend, they post photos of themselves to their group. What's next? They see this program does work and they ask the questions: What's next for me? What can I build now?"

"We encourage exchanges between beginners and those who've gone down the road a little," says Joan. "Like me. They look at me and how far I've come. I became the 'it girl' of the older generation! To be that girl and getting accolades from strangers—all I wanted to do was turn it around, pass it on. There's a way of eating and training we were never taught. What if everybody were able to take care of themselves? What about strength instead of fixing what's broken? It's a much better quality of life."

WHAT TO DO WHEN ...

Getting discouraged is part of anything we do in life. But *becoming* discouraged and *staying* discouraged are two different things.

Focusing on your new to-do list will help. Reminding yourself of the whys and the hows of your new lifestyle is essential. Some people like keeping a photograph on their phone to show them where they want to go. Some apps also include motivational sections. Michelle also recommends the Marc & Angel website (www.marcandangel.com) for quick, positive self-talk in bite-sized bits.

"I'm so enticed by life. There's so much to see, so much to enjoy if you just take the time. That saying about stopping to smell the roses, it's so apt. Enjoy your life, every moment, because you can be sure that someone out there is having a worse time than you even could ever think of. Appreciate what you have. I tell that to myself all the time. Some people can't walk and you're worried about not feeling good? You're moaning about how it hurts to do the exercises? Some people have no sensation—they'd love to hurt.
Keep things in perspective!"

CONSISTENCY & SCHEDULING

When it comes to working out, there's no magic number of days or hours you need to hit the gym. What's most important is being consistent. If you can only commit to three days a week, make sure you stick with it and don't skip any workouts. You'll get better benefits from a long-term program that works with your lifestyle. Each week's little progress adds up to big results.

Over time, you can gradually increase the frequency and duration of your workouts. Remember, even 20 minutes of exercise can make a difference, so if you can't fit in a long workout, don't sweat it. Just do what you can and be consistent with it.

"Gym wasn't part and parcel of my life before," says Joan. "Now when I miss going, I'm lost! Keeping to a schedule means staying on track. Simple things. Having my meals every three hours. When I get off track, it's usually because something's cut into the time. I try to be prepared all the time, but sometimes, it just wobbles. Then I go back to the basics. As long as you get those meals in and space them out."

That preparation Joan talks about is all in the planning, the scheduling—whether it's for meals, weight training, or just going for a walk. "Before and after workouts are the largest meals. My first meal is a substantial meal that hits the macros. Then I feel better for the rest of the day."

And it's not just about eating. Sleep is an essential consideration. "I have my workout in the morning so the rest of the day I can get everything else done. I'm in bed by 9 p.m. or even before that because I get up early and I want to get eight hours of sleep at least. In fact, my body is even happier with more! My body has a cycle. I don't set an alarm anymore. I just wake up between 5:30 and 6 a.m."

She recognizes that there's effort involved. "A lot of time management is necessary to stay on track," Joan says. "But think about it: You do your work at an office on schedule, don't you? So what's different about this? Your work is a serious business. You can enjoy it, sure, but you don't joke around either. So all the more reason you don't want to joke around with your health. It's serious business too."

None of that time management falls into place automatically. Consistency and scheduling are learned behaviors, and the sooner you get into the habit of managing how and where you spend your time, the easier the whole process will be. And as we said at the beginning of this book: The way to start is to just start.

"If you really want to do this, move!" says Joan. "Move right now. If you're sitting around watching TV, turn it off, get up. Once you've started moving, you'll find a lot of the rest falls into place. Some people are naturally disorganized. That's okay, but you've got to do a lot of change within if you want to have a big change in your life.

"Be serious about it. Not to the point of not being fun—but seriously all the same. This is your life we're talking about. If you want your health, you have to work for it. You can't buy it or get it back. Anything worthwhile, you have to work for. It doesn't just drop in your lap. I still have to put in the effort."

WHAT'S A TYPICAL DAY LIKE FOR JOAN?

"I get up early," Joan says. "The first thing I do is some deep breathing. Then I do my journaling and maybe answer some questions on the Train with Joan app or the Journal with Joan app. Then I give myself some time practicing my Spanish with Duolingo and a little more time on Elevate, an app that exercises your brain. By now it's 7 a.m."

That means time for breakfast and then she's off to the gym. She works out, showers, then has her postworkout meal. "Hopefully, I don't have any correspondence other than Instagram, so the rest of my day flows around my eating every three hours. I do my shopping, banking, all those errands during the day. And, of course, I spend more time answering questions on Instagram—it's really easy to get lost there, so I try to break it up some, do it for an hour, and then go for a coffee."

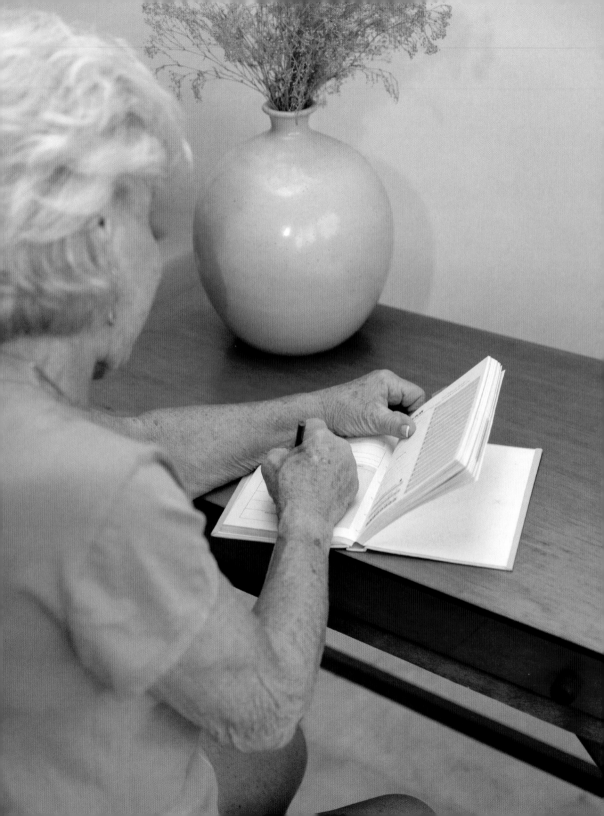

Supper is at 5:30 p.m. "Generally after that, I'm on some call or another, a journaling group, a The Wonder Women group. And in my own group, there are assignments to complete and communication with the other girls in training. We share recipes, talk about podcasts that are helpful, respond to questions the coach brings up. I get to bed by 9 p.m. at the latest. I need my beauty sleep!"

Joan works out at the gym five days a week. Two of those days are for high-intensity cardio training; the other three for isolating different body parts and working with weights. "I like to be outside," she says, "so I often do some of my long cardio cycling around. It's a half hour down to the beach, maybe a swim, then a half hour back. That will give you a good workout for sure!"

WHAT DREAMS CAN YOU REACH FOR NOW?

Joan says that possibly the best part of transformation is how it's changed the way she sees herself. "I wasn't a person who took chances," she says. "Now I can't wait to see what's coming next!

"Ask yourself: What was your intention to begin with? What are your hopes? You have to focus on that because anything that's going to change is going to take time. You can spend time doing nothing or you can spend that time doing something for yourself even if you don't want to go through the whole process. Be honest: Do you really want to make a better life for yourself and can you take all the criticisms that will go with it? If I don't do it, I have nothing to fight with. If anything does happen, I have ammunition. If that's not what you want, I can't help. That effort has to come from the person."

Reaching for the stars just isn't possible when you're in a place of tiredness, of low self-esteem, of discouragement. But isn't that what our lives—at their brightest and best—should be aiming for? To fill our lives in as much as we can with wondrous things, daring activities, challenging opportunities, ways we can impact our lives and those around us in a positive and edifying way?

Look again at your goals. They might have changed since you started reading this book or used the Train with Joan app or you might feel even more strongly that the ones you started with are still the best for you right now.

Perhaps it's just the language that needs to change. Think of the two different kinds of goals. A "push" goal is one you have to—wait for it—push to complete. It has to get done and chances are you don't want to do it for myriad possible reasons. Push goals are more difficult to attain because you have to constantly use your willpower to even take a step in the right direction. A "pull" goal is one you feel drawn to. You want it. You spend a lot of time thinking about it. Instead of constantly pushing you, a pull goal is one you're eager to work toward. It's all about enthusiasm—and even passion.

You won't feel motivated all the time, but if you're driven by your passion to give yourself the gift of a vibrant, healthy lifestyle, then your goals will feel like something you want to claim for yourself.

"I feel like I have clear direction and goals that have expanded beyond fitness into other areas of my life," says one The Wonder Women participant. "I'm excited for life and truly feel like the sky's the limit!"

Joan has certainly found that her transformation journey opened up far more to her than she'd ever dreamed of. "I have a bucket list, but I'm open to trying anything!" she says. What's on the list?

"Oh, let's see. I want to visit England and stay for a while—enough time to really get to know the place and the people. I'd love to meet up with people who follow me there. And a European river cruise. And Australia! Before I met my husband, I considered emigrating to Australia. We have some gals all over the world. Wouldn't it be fun to visit and meet them in their home countries? I'd love to find someone younger and adventurous as a traveling companion, someone to go along and maybe keep an eye on me, someone who loves to travel and do new things!"

One thing I can say is that really getting to a place where you've fine-tuned the needs of your body for optimal functioning and getting to a place of truly robust health and longevity are worthwhile pursuits for all of us.

Michelle MacDonald

And it's not all about travel either. "Yes, I'm a lot more daring now," she admits. "I'd try parachuting or skydiving, although maybe not bungee jumping because of my shoulder. You have to know your limitations. I'd love to go white water rafting too. I've never done that. And more kayaking. I went scuba diving for the first time. It was great. I was supposed to go with two younger gals and they backed out. Can you imagine? I've become the family daredevil! Entertainment parks are my playground. Ferris wheels used to scare me, but now they attract me. As I look back, I think I was always a daredevil, but it didn't manifest itself until I got into shape. Now I really want to go places and do things. I really want to shine for myself. I always had that in me, but it took this transformation of my lifestyle to allow it to come out."

Her enthusiasm is infectious. "Sometimes, I think there's not enough time to do everything I want to do—I feel like I'm just getting started," Joan says. "What I want to say to people is this: Go for it. New opportunities are always opening up to you. Get a little excited. Break out of your shell. Life is so much exciting when you're out of your comfort zone. Just try!"

Kim Falconer

I was alive—but not living life. I had no excitement for the future. Then I saw Joan's transformation and it was different. She emitted a zeal for life and spark that let others know they could change. I watched her daughter Michelle, and together, they intrigued me. They showed passion for their lifestyle. They truly wanted to help others. I realized I wouldn't age healthy unless I changed.

My weight was at an all-time high and my self-esteem at an all-time low. In our program, we took weekly check-in photos. I struggled to look at the camera. Initially, I barely saw change. At three months, I realized Michelle's program was molding my body and mind. I started to believe the positive words others were saying to me. I didn't yet believe in myself. At six months, I began to believe in myself and talk kindly to myself. I'd been prediabetic with high cholesterol. I started the program with what I thought was arthritis in my back and a weak knee from a past surgery. Today, my cholesterol is normal, my blood shows I'm no longer prediabetic, I don't feel like I have arthritis, and I no longer have a weak knee. This journey has been a miracle that has helped me change directions emotionally and physically. I'm excited to age gracefully. This journey has changed those around me. My husband started exercising with me and changed the direction his health was heading. My sister-in-law has started weight training. My children and their spouses have all joined gyms. The list goes on. I see how Joan and Michelle caused a ripple effect.

Michelle and Joan are changing lives one woman at a time. My hope is to help others see that all they need to do is start and each day try to do a little better. Time will pass no matter what. Build healthy habits. Learn what you need for you and keep those as nonnegotiables. Talk kindly to yourself—you deserve that! Don't compare yourself with others. Celebrate you and your wins, even the smallest ones. One day, like me, you'll no longer recognize the person in the application photo. You'll see the girl you were long ago oozing out as you skip, laugh, and find joy in your day-to-day life. My life is forever changed.

CHAPTER SEVEN:

FINDING YOUR COMMUNITY

My team of 20 became my second family. These women understood. They got me. The texts each morning, the group calls, the encouraging words underneath our weekly photo collages–each one was like glue holding all the pieces together. To be a Wonder Women member is truly an empowering experience.

The Wonder Women participant

You can't go it alone.

That's the message from Joan and Michelle as well as women who've participated in The Wonder Women and women who use the Train with Joan app. There's a reason Michelle and Joan have become Instagram influencers: They not only understand the need for community, but they also put in the time and effort necessary to "be there" for tens of thousands of others. "I'm on the app every day," says Joan, "even though the technology's still not easy for me. But it's also incredible how many people you can reach. Who would've ever thought so many people would know my name, that I'd become an important part of their lives? And most of them are gals I'll never meet. But if I can help them stay motivated, that's why I'm there. It's for the community."

The medical establishment recognizes the need for others to help us stay motivated. "Relying on willpower is a frequent recipe for failure, as it's a limited resource and is easily overwhelmed by stress, fatigue, or even enjoyment of things we know aren't necessarily 'good for us,'" says Dr. Cedric X. Bryant, chief science officer at the American Council on Exercise.

"Social support from friends, family, coworkers, and other important players in your life can be a strong predictor of how successful you will be in adhering to a behavior change over the long term."

So it stands to reason that even when just preparing to undergo any kind of lifestyle transformation, you create a supportive community *a priori*. There are many different ways of finding community, of creating that support system you need for success. You can choose to follow a transformational program that includes community as one of its pillars. That's what Joan and Michelle find works best.

"I want to give a shout-out to all the beautiful women out there who not only decide to make a change but who also help others light their torch," says Joan. "The more we all pick up the reins and charge forth, spreading positivity and good, factual information about health and wellness, the better."

But even if you're part of a program with a built-in community, you'll still need to have others in your sphere "on your side," so to speak. People who are behind you as you reach for your goals. People who'll celebrate milestones with you, listen when you need to talk about your journey, and provide inspiration when your energy might be dwindling.

For some, that support can be built in through their families. "My husband told me when I applied that he'd do anything he could to help me," says one program participant. "He accompanied me to every single workout. He did bench presses, squats, and booty band lifts with my pink and purple bands right next to me, never once complaining. My heart swells when I think about how much he supported me throughout this."

On the other hand, Joan's husband "wouldn't be caught dead in a gym!" But her daughter and son-in-law are cheering her on every day.

Social support can take a lot of different forms and those various aspects might not all be delivered by the same individual or community. You might find your inspirational support in one place, practical support in another, and emotional support in a third. Everybody's life is different.

The one caveat? Where you find your community is optional, but having that community isn't.

"You have to surround yourself with the people you need," stresses Joan. "Sometimes, that means making different friends. It's like when people go into Alcoholics Anonymous. Sometimes, to stay sober, they just can't keep hanging out with the same people they were with before—people who aren't living the life they want."

But it's also about having fun in the process. "This is all about getting healthy," says Joan. "And that means trying new things too. Find someone to do things with, go on adventures with as a group. No one wants to do new things alone. Everything's much more fun when you share it with others."

Instagram played a big role in establishing Joan's own community and out of it grew the Train with Joan app that touches and helps so many people. "Instagram is a great platform for getting out information," Joan says. "I'm always blown away by how many followers I have. I wasn't planning on anything like that, but my daughter felt that because I was an introvert—you wouldn't believe that, would you?— it would be a good way to communicate with people, share the journey I'm on, and help them on theirs. By the end of the first year, I had a couple thousand followers and it's just taken off since then.

"Of course, when I make a post, it's usually the same people who are the first to respond! I recognize them, so I have this ongoing connection. And I try to respond to everyone. It's a job that keeps me busy many hours of the day. I've had posts where there were between 5,000 and 8,000 responses! Even just to read their names takes hours, let alone responding. And if they've asked an actual question, I feel I have to respond to them. I can't leave these people hanging. I've spent hours with my eyes hurting from looking at the screen, but it's so worth it. It's everything!"

CREATING A SUPPORT STRUCTURE & GETTING THE SUPPORT YOU NEED

If you're not part of an intense program, such as The Wonder Women, then you'll need to be creative about giving yourself as many options for support as you can. These options might change throughout your transformation—people move away, you might change gyms, you might simply find that someone isn't giving you the help you need—but never drop any of it until you've found a replacement.

The structure of your community is up to you. Creating a community? That's a nonnegotiable.

Community brings in more benefits than you might think. The support your community gives you isn't a one-way street. Just as the individuals in your group are there for you, you're also there for them. Yes, that's altruistic, but the truth is, it feels good to help someone else! Seeing yourself as a role model for others and helping them along their journey reaffirms you're on the right road.

"At first, I was leery of people at the gym," says Joan. "But those same people, they're the ones who ended up supporting me. They'd say something like, 'Wow, your shoulders are great.' I'd remember hearing that and what it meant to me, to feel part of this thing that everyone's there doing together, taking care of your health. So I started telling people too when I'd see positive changes in them. It's like an affirmation circle."

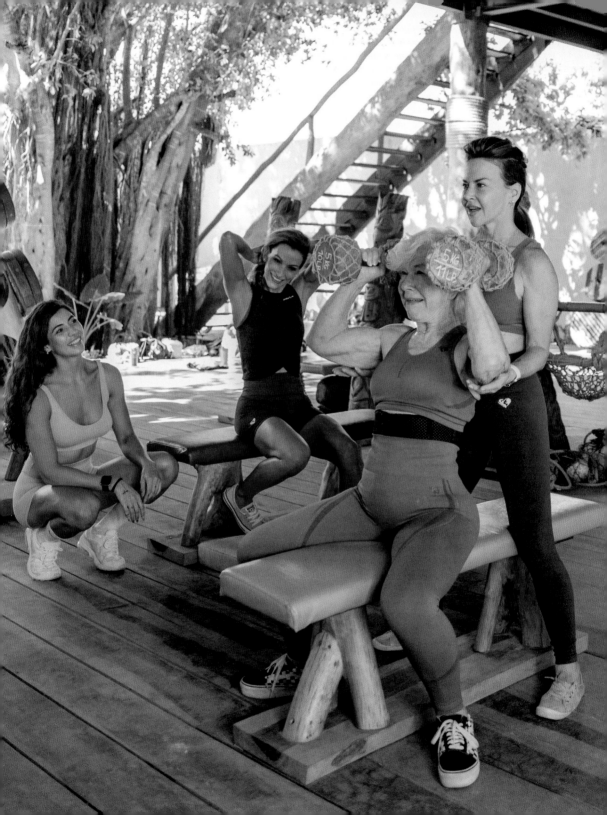

And it doesn't just help with exercise. "There's so much autonomy in meal planning with macros that it's absolutely huge to have a community where you can share all these ways of doing it—a place where you can take pride in your meal planning," says Michelle.

The community you create is your community, so pick the people you want to have there. "I've been lucky in choosing friends," Joan admits. "I didn't have any who were negative about my process. I want to have people around me who I can rely on. It's true that if you only have a few true friends, it's better than having tons of fair-weather friends."

So as you think about building your own community, your first step is to figure out what kind of support you need. What will not just keep you on track but also keep you motivated and inspired and positive? Remember, one person or even one organization might not be able to fulfill all your needs. It's up to you to get creative and put together a program that works.

IDENTIFYING YOUR NEEDS

What kind of support will best help you navigate your transformation? Think about your needs as you consider who to include in your community. A supportive community will help you address problems and it will be there for you when you're feeling stress, discouragement, or any other negative feelings that pop up along the way. Sitting alone with those feelings can make you feel trapped inside them, but sharing them with others opens the door to allow them to flow through you and escape—and replace them with affirmations and support.

That sharing opens up a flow of communication and caring. It's hard to change behaviors. Joan and Michelle agree on that. "I'm honest with people: It's not easy," says Michelle. "You have to really want it." Feelings of stress or other negative factors can interfere with your dedication and determination. This is where support from your team comes in. They help you remember your goals, remind you of your triumphs, and exhibit empathy around your challenges—just as you'd turn around and do for them too. One The Wonder Women participant found the camaraderie of the community a major asset. "We fueled our health goals by focusing on finding joy in our process," she says. "And slowly but surely, our metrics and mindsets began to change."

For metrics and mindsets to change, you first need to find a way to stay on track. What that means is sticking with the program, allowing for the occasional lapse, but getting back on it. So the first thing you need to consider is accountability.

You're not alone! There are groups that provide accountability for all sorts of goals. Some groups require daily or even hourly check-ins to report plans and then note whether members followed through on those specific plans—be it for an hour, a day, or a week. Everything from professional tasks to religious reminders is available.

This move toward accountability is popular for one great reason: It works. Telling someone you're going to do something and then having to face them afterward might be just the incentive some of us need to keep going. The embarrassment of not reporting success might not be a positive motivator, but it can work to your advantage.

The success of programs like Alcoholics Anonymous, which provides support and accountability to individuals addicted to alcohol, points to the truth behind the organization's structure: As social creatures, we don't do very well on our own when we're trying to effect transformation.

Whether that transformation entails abstention from something or changing the way one views food and exercise, it's essential to reflect your progress and your problems back to other people—whether you're looking for counsel and advice or just a witness to your endeavor.

So what do you need? You've come this far in the book, which means you've identified your decision to transform your body—and, with it, your life. You've learned some fundamental truths about fitness and nutrition. You've considered motivation and preparing yourself for a brand-new chapter in your story. Let's break down what might be included in your particular needs for support:

- **Emotional.** Change takes time, but we humans tend to reach for immediate gratification. Sometimes, you just don't feel like doing your program. That's when you need encouragement to help you get through the "not feeling it today" syndrome.

- **Accountable.** Setting a goal is great, but reaching it is even better. If you keep your goals to yourself, then you can tend to gloss over the ones you don't reach. "I'll do it tomorrow—it doesn't matter." But if at the end of the day you need to check in with someone about that day's specific plans or goals, then you're far more likely to achieve them.

- **Practical.** Sometimes, the difference between getting to the gym and not getting to the gym might be as simple as finding someone to mind your kids for an hour and a half. Or maybe you've been at home caring for a sick child and couldn't get to the grocery store to buy what you need to stick to your nutrition plan. Is there someone willing to make a shopping run for you? This kind of support is often overlooked, but it's invaluable.

- **Inspirational.** One of the phrases we've encountered throughout this book is "If she can do it, I can do it!" Joan has been an inspiration for countless women who are now living healthy, vital, engaged lives. Find her on Instagram and download her app—and you have instant inspiration. Finding additional role models will only underscore the effect. Maybe there's someone at your gym you really look up to—a trainer or another "gym rat," as Joan calls them. Just watching their form and commitment can make you become determined to reach higher. Inspirational support can also be that friend who commits to working out with you, encourages you to keep moving, and helps you stay motivated to stick to your goals. She might send you cards with helpful quotes on them. She might collect success stories to share with you. She might remind you in myriad ways that she believes in you and is expecting you to be successful.

So as you think about your community, make sure you tick off all the boxes. It's not expected that the same person will provide all the different avenues of support you need. That's not what community is about! But if you have your specific needs and goals in mind, you'll be best equipped to find the right group or individuals to help you claim the life you're aiming for.

As you think about forming a support system for yourself, remember that most people aren't mind readers. "A lot of folks just assume that their family and friends will see what their needs are and will step in to fill them," says Joan. "It just doesn't work that way. It's up to every one of us to ask for what we need."

When you do, be specific. "I'm going to need your support" is a nice phrase, but it's ultimately meaningless. Everyone will nod and commit to being supportive—that's easy. But being there for the emotional meltdowns, the hard slogging, the myriad details real support involves is a lot more difficult.

Let's take a couple examples:

1. You've committed to your macro-based nutrition program. It's been designed by your coach or nutritionist with your specific needs in mind. You feel great about it. Two or three weeks in, your friend Carol wants to take you out to lunch. Eventually, you'll get to a point where you can analyze foods in restaurants and make choices that stay within your parameters, but right now, it's too soon for that. Carol might mean well, but she's sabotaging your plan. Worse still, if you refuse, she might be offended. How do you tell her she isn't being supportive when she thinks she is?

2. Your friend Rachel works out at your gym. She's a treadmill fiend. You've committed to building muscle mass and want to spend most of your workout times lifting weights. Rachel complains that when you do go to the gym together, she never sees you and wonders what the point is of even going together.

The only way to circumvent these situations and others like them is to be very clear when you tell your family and friends about what you're doing and be equally clear with those you'll be asking for help. "I'm not going to be able to eat out for a while" is a good way to warn people that a restaurant lunch is off the table, so to speak. You can still figure out ways of incorporating your friendships into your program. For example, you can meet Carol for a walk around the lake instead of for lunch.

So be specific. Replace "Can you help with carpooling?" with "Would you be able to drop Melinda off at choir practice on Thursdays?" Replace "I'm on a diet" with "I'm eating according to a personalized nutrition plan."

FINDING YOUR COMMUNITY— ONLINE & OFF

One of the positive results of the technological revolution is how communicating with the world has become simple and almost thoughtless. Where once upon a time people waited for letters to arrive, carrying on conversations that took place over weeks if not months (or even years!), now those conversations can be held in real time.

The Wonder Women program is completely online. Participants need to access Zoom to talk with their groups and use phone/tablet apps for information about and recording of macros, meal plans, weight training, and exercise examples and logs.

At the other end of the spectrum from that fully online interaction are those people whose analog worlds are far more developed, important, and comfortable than their internet-based ones. They prefer conversations in which all participants are in the same room—literally. They'd rather have a cup of tea with a friend than hop on a Zoom call.

For many of us, life is lived somewhere between the two extremes. What matters isn't your mode of getting to community. What matters is that you do it. "I always say to join a community of like-minded women," says Joan, "even if it's online! And make an effort to connect meaningfully. Help others. Ask for help."

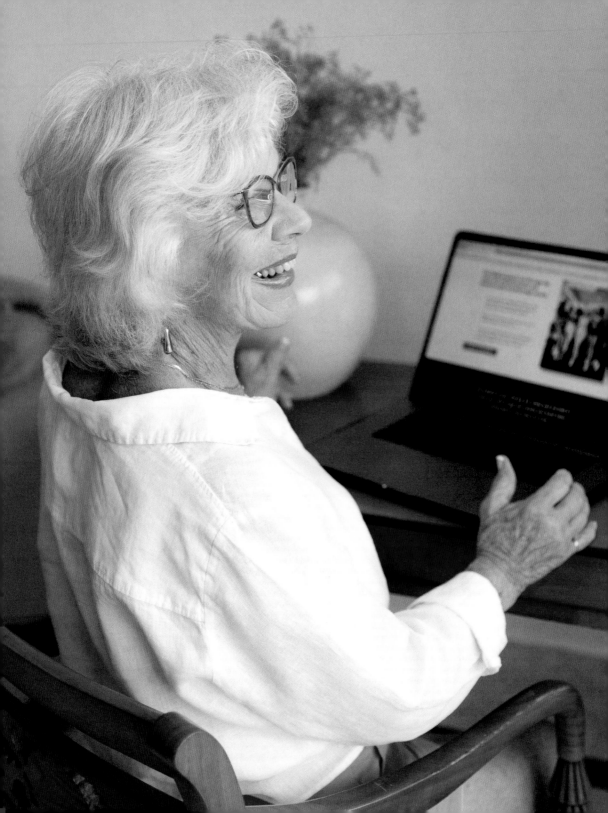

CREATING A COMMUNITY

You might find that none of the available options are best for you. Perhaps you're finding it difficult to talk about your journey with strangers. Maybe a support group's meeting times just haven't worked out for you. Or you might just want to do something hyperlocal in your own neighborhood or town. A friend might be talking about having similar goals as yours.

There's no reason why you can't start a support group of your own. After all, people start book clubs, money management groups, even accountability teams. Why not create your own community?

If you do want to start your own group, make sure you're all agreed from the start on a series of fundamental choices:

- **When to meet.** Keeping a regular day and time is helpful.

- **Where to meet.** Decide whether this is online, offline, or a hybrid.

- **How often to meet.** Consistency is key to making sure you're getting together often enough.

- **Group size.** You might start small and then increase the size over time once everyone sees how things go with a small group.

- **Structure.** Is one person in charge? Who'll send out the invites?

- **Goals.** These are for the group and/or for the individuals.

- **How to spend your time together.** Having an agenda or a set program for each meeting can help keep everyone focused.

- **Getting expert help.** Will you invite professionals, such as trainers or nutritionists, to speak? How will you pay for that?

Be supportive! It's not enough to share your journey itself. This is where you can bring challenges and triumphs alike. Facing a particular challenge? Your group can help you figure out a solution. Feeling discouraged? This is where you'll get your pep talks. Want to share something that really worked and motivate others to try it too? Bring it! Start a recipe-sharing circle, show each other photos, write your goals and aspirations in a chat group thread or on a whiteboard.

For this community to work, it's important that every group member feels invested in each other's success. You're all in it together. When one of you shares a success, a milestone moment, a compliment she received, it's as if it happened to you too. This is one of the great joys of community.

A community doesn't necessarily have to be a group per se. Try to find several people willing to provide what you might call "emergency support": ways of helping you talk yourself down off a ledge when you're feeling discouraged or vulnerable. As you get more experienced and have some success under your belt, consider providing that same emergency help to others. The best way to build community is for it to be a give-and-take situation.

FOLLOWING A PROGRAM VS. GOING IT ALONE

Obviously, Joan and Michelle feel that following a program has remarkable advantages over making significant lifestyle choices and changes on your own. There are many reasons for this, starting with the fact of The Wonder Women being a program that has been tested and honed and delivers success. In addition, though, it and many other programs can offer tremendous benefits, such as:

- access to experts
- instant community
- education
- supervision
- effective techniques
- personalization
- detailed guidelines

On the other hand, there are also some excellent reasons for not joining a group/program such as The Wonder Women. The first is the cost. We freely admit that's a barrier for many. Some women find they can't fit an intensive program with tightly scheduled meetings into their professional and/or home lives. Others, for various reasons, just aren't able to join a lifestyle transformation group.

So for some, designing your own program might be the best (and possibly only) option.

DESIGNING YOUR OWN PROGRAM

First and foremost, as we've said elsewhere, it's essential you consult with an expert at a minimum to set up your program. Everyone has different specific health situations and a certified trainer and nutritionist can take your health needs as well as your preferences into account to design a program that's safe and functional for your life requirements and goals. It's always a good idea to check with your primary physician before starting any kind of program—whether group or individual—to make sure all your health needs are taken into account.

That said, you can have a group in which individual members have their own goals, meal plans, and exercise programs but still meet together to give each other support, exchange information, or even eat and/or exercise together.

Any good program should include the following:

- **Establishing a nutrition program.** Try to balance every meal for protein, fat, and carbohydrates. Besides the right nutrients, eating the right foods at the right time can help your body make the most of the exercise you're doing and see better results.

- **Training with weights.** Not only does weight training burn a large number of calories in the gym, but increased muscle tone and size also give you a higher metabolic rate, even when you're asleep. Weight training appears to maintain lean body weight more effectively than aerobic exercise.

- **Incorporating cardiovascular exercise.** Although probably not as crucial as weight training for fat loss, cardio still plays a critical role. To get your body to burn your fat stores, exercise at low intensities and for longer periods of time. Lower intensities use the fat-burning, aerobic, slow-twitch muscle fibers for force production to a high degree.

- **Trying for slow weight loss.** Losing weight faster than 1 to 2 pounds a week will increase the amount of weight you lose from lean tissue and body water and decrease pounds lost from fat.

- **Drinking plenty of water.** Staying hydrated will help your body function at its best and can reduce fatigue. Aim to drink three to five liters of water per day. "Don't worry: Your body adjusts to it," says Joan. "At first, it feels like you're always going to the washroom! But your body adjusts."

Applying all these principles—individually and in your group—can help everyone stay on track. And it makes trying something new a lot less intimidating. One of the Wonder Women participants confessed: "Almost all the exercises were new to me and the 'bro gym' was incredibly intimidating. I didn't know how to set up a tripod and actually record myself doing these lifts. What if I looked stupid? What if I had no idea how to set up the bar? What if? What if? What if?"

But she didn't give up because she had the support and weight of her community behind her. And you can too.

USING YOUR COMMUNITY TO STAY MOTIVATED

Modeling any community on others that have been successful can be helpful. The example we keep returning to is, of course, The Wonder Women. Through trial and error, Michelle has created a program that just works. And a large part of its success is in the community, the friendships, and the support these women share. They in turn look to encourage others.

One The Wonder Women participant explains: "Now I have a heart and a passion to help that woman who's struggling. The one who can't get out of bed. The one who feels like 'Those days are past' and she'll never look like she did before. The one who hurts all over and is at an increased risk of breaking a bone. The one who emotionally eats because food has been the only thing that has consistently ever been there for her. I hope one day to help her."

A supportive social network can empower and enable you to address problems and provide emotional support when feelings of stress or other negative factors threaten to interfere with your quest to make behavioral changes. Another benefit of social support is that it's a two-way street: You're providing that support in addition to receiving it. "Knowing that I'm keeping all these gals motivated keeps me motivated," says Joan.

There's no question it can feel lonely when you're changing your life in radical ways and your friends and family might find themselves a little baffled by your dedication. They don't understand the commitment.

They don't even speak the same language as you do when describing what you're doing. That's where this very specific community comes in.

"The community is like an incredible, global sisterhood," says Joan. "I've had so much fun with these women and you know it's not easy to find people who really get the journey you are on. With these gals, it's like finding instant best friends and no one bats an eye when you talk about macros or getting your steps in or buying a new hip thrust pad!"

Eventually, your community is the group that will see you through the challenges, triumphs, setbacks, and joys that come with transforming your current life into something vibrant, healthy, and much happier. "You have to change the way you think about yourself," Joan adds. "When you do, that spills over into other people. No one's perfect. Some people aren't demonstrative, for example. But sometimes, when you feel negative about someone, you later find out they really admired you—but couldn't tell you. When you see someone who has that problem, you naturally want to help them transform. There's a ripple effect going on. I have a friend back in my old town, when she's at the coffee shop drive-through, she pays for the person behind her. A lot of people do the pay-it-forward thing. If we all take care of each other, I think the rest will take care of itself."

Cheryl Sparks

Stuck. Depressed. Achy. Cranky. Broken. That's how I felt as I scrolled Instagram. It was yet another day I couldn't pull myself out of bed. Another day I asked, "What does it matter anyway?" Then a white-haired lady popped up on my screen. She was *ripped*. Watching her do overhead presses, my jaw went slack. But most of all, it was her smile. She truly looked joyous, vibrant.

Who was this woman? How did she get here? As the weeks went by, I couldn't get Joan out of my head. If she could do this, why couldn't I? I decided then that I was in. I joined the Train with Joan program. Every time Joan popped up on my app, I grinned—and set my jaw in determination.

When I got started with The Wonder Women, little did I know how much my mindset would also be strengthened! How emotional and mental fitness would play an even larger role in my change. I became more aware of how much I was limiting myself in my mind, which was, in turn, stunting any kind of personal growth I attempted.

It wasn't until about the 90-day mark that people around me started commenting. To me, I was seeing changes, but no one was saying anything. Suddenly, one day, it happened. A few people who hadn't seen me for a few months literally didn't recognize me. "Oh my goodness! What *are* you doing? You look *fantastic*!"

My life was back. My smile matched Joan's. I now glow. My mental energy is no longer spent on trying on four different outfits each morning, throwing them on the floor in disgust. My emotional strength is rock solid. I self-coach myself daily–throughout stressful times at work, when I feel myself getting anxious and wanting to dive headfirst into a vat of Reese's Peanut Butter Cups, when I hear that old voice popping up saying, "Does it even matter anyway?" Because, yes. Yes, it does matter. I matter. There are people out there who need the best version of Cheryl possible.

I'm eternally grateful for Michelle and Joan. For Joan's courage to embark on such an incredible and difficult path of changing her life. For Michelle's love for her mom and for starting a program that would change the worlds of those who choose to follow it. I have a toolbox full of knowledge, journals, training logs, recipes, and friends to help keep me on my path as I move forward, continuing to spiral upward.

CONCLUSION

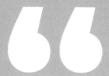

No one is going to hand you your greatness. You've got to earn that stuff every damn day with your grit, your joy, your wit, and your optimism.

Michelle MacDonald

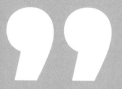

"I used to have a mantra," says Joan. "I don't use it much anymore, but it was really helpful when I was starting out on my journey. It's this: You're a gift from the Lord. God gave you this life—make the most of it. Make it better if you can. Above all, don't waste it."

Many people—especially women—feel at some point like they've compromised their best interests over time and end up looking at themselves in a mirror and wondering, "What happened?"

Joan has an answer: "Life happened," she says. "But you can change it around. Just try some of the things I've talked about here: eating better, working your brain, getting up, and doing things. It doesn't have to be workouts as such—just get moving. Guard your sleep. It's precious. Drink a lot of water. It only takes a little bit of effort. I wish more people could be healthier—and they can!"

Mindset is a dominant part of becoming healthier. "You have to change the story," says Joan. "Stop feeling sorry for yourself. There are no easy answers to anything in life. You have to own your mistakes and that's a hard pill to swallow, but you feel better when you do something about it."

Recognizing your feelings and analyzing your actions will take insight and mindfulness.

It's far easier sometimes to just put yourself on autopilot, to just go through the motions. "Hours later, you'll try to remember whether you did something," says Joan. "What happened between this and this? That's not mindful. It's great when you know exactly what you're doing at what time. When you don't, when you don't think about yourself in the moment, then you miss so much in life. I know what it's like to go on autopilot. I did it myself for a long time. I don't ever want to do that again."

She's certainly not on autopilot these days. "When I'm working out, I focus on what I'm doing, on all the cues I've been given, and I hope I don't forget anything. Someone said to me recently: 'You look so serious when you're working out. You're not smiling.' That's because I'm concentrating on what I'm doing. I'm thinking about it. I'm in the moment," Joan says.

And that focus, that mindfulness, that dedication can be anyone's. You don't have to be young or fit or anything special. You just have to want it. You just have to internally set your clock for the new you and start asking yourself what wonderful things you'll be able to accomplish and enjoy when you're that person, when you've found your *why*.

"Anyone can do it," says Michelle. "Anyone can transform. Look at my mother. She got off her medications. She got two decades back— more really because she's better than she was at 56. Mom isn't a one-shot wonder. She's still my oldest client, but her transformation isn't unique."

Being "better" is a goal everyone can set because "fitness" is going to look different for different people. But everyone can become better versions of themselves. Everyone can grow. Everyone can build something new and lasting.

It's what Michelle believes—and has proven time and time again. "I just look at my mom, at the joy of trying new things, of making new friends in your 70s. Fitness isn't a goal in itself unless you really twist things—

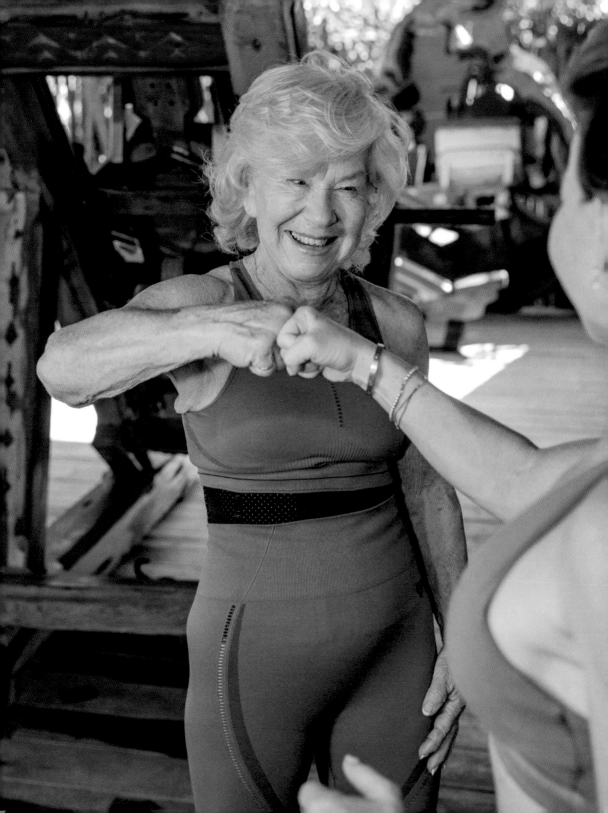

it's about enjoying your life to the fullest. The habits and behaviors you'll learn are positive. They build character. People become more organized, they're calmer, they have better relationships, they're more aware. All these things are such tangible rewards and are available to everybody. Anyone can achieve that kind of lifestyle. It's just out there, waiting for you. You're creating a new reality based on your shift in identity: from believing in yourself to doing the small daily things that lead up to those big wins."

Today, Joan is an Instagram influencer with followers all over the planet. "On every continent but Antarctica," she likes to say. She's a role model for women of all ages. She shares her thoughts and changes people's lives. "When I was a kid, I'd listen to adults— sometimes when they didn't know I was there. It's interesting what you can learn by just listening. Listening is an art. A lot of people are talking without saying anything. I'm quiet with people because I want to get a feel of where they're coming from. I don't want to talk and have nothing to say. I wish more people would listen." When it's Joan talking, it's fair to say there are plenty of listeners.

For Michelle, it's also about listening—to what your heart is telling you. "But then you have to commit," she says. It's not just your heart but also your mind you'll need to engage. "Going at your own pace—that's pop psychology," she says. "Get in, get out. You can lose 30 pounds in 4 months. It's within your reach. Get your focus aligned, get clarity around what you're doing, hit those early targets—that's what will keep you motivated—and achieve the goal, then switch to maintenance and principles of reverse dieting.

"Don't miss the boat. Don't take too long. Find out what you can do— and do it. Don't do just the minimum. You have to have some quick success to keep the flame lit. The coach in me makes me say that. You don't want to get distracted. Immerse yourself in this lifestyle. But for sure commit to regular training, even if just four exercises a day. Commit to a 10-minute walk before each meal. Get a lot of stuff in the 'I did this right' bucket. That shift in identity is essential. Keep your passion burning around the *why* and you can't go wrong."

"There's always that temptation to go back," says Joan. "A smell will bring up a memory that's enticing, even though you know it's not good for you. You just have to leave it alone. I keep thinking about why I wanted to start this in the first place and I don't want any part of how I was back then. I just want to live a healthy life, enjoy what I can."

She's received a plethora of letters from daughters who saw her online and encouraged their mothers to apply the program's principles, "and they turned their mothers into a functioning person," says Joan. "One woman lived in a nursing home, where she barely shuffled around. She couldn't even turn a door handle. Once she started getting proper food and doing some exercises, she improved. Within a year, she was walking two blocks, putting on her own clothing, eating properly. She wouldn't have gone through that transformation if I hadn't first gone through mine."

What does Joan hope readers will take away from this book? "What's important is being healthy and passing on what you learn to others," she says. "If each reader got just one other person to do something, that ripple effect is the most beneficial to getting the word out. You don't have to do exactly what I did, but do something. Don't say you can't until you've given it a really good shot."

And it's not complicated. "If you don't do it on the inside, you'll lose it. Because you don't know how to talk yourself into something positive. I've seen it happen too many times. I like going to the fitness shows, seeing the person transform. All I want is health. If the rest follows, that's a bonus. But I'd sooner change the inner person. Love yourself. Then you won' t throw it all away.

"Just keep trying," says Joan. "And keep doing what you really want to do, what you really love doing. Don't say you can't do it. Don't say you can't have it. You deserve some love and laughter in your life, and that doesn't end when you're 40 or 50. You can have joy and happiness until the day you die."

Joanne Zimmerman

I taught Bikram yoga, went to yoga training, started teaching it—and heard about Michelle. I started following her. I saw all she was accomplishing with weightlifting and following a bodybuilder lifestyle. Seeing how she had developed a completely different physique fascinated me. While I'm open to trying new things, I'd never tried weightlifting before.

The years were getting on and I wasn't thrilled about how I was aging, how I was feeling about my strength and body composition. Something was missing. Then I saw Joan's transformation and I thought, "Why wouldn't I do this?" Joan was achieving goals at her age. I saw the incredible muscle she was developing and it made me think I could do it too. I applied, did the program, and my group really became sisters in so many ways. We each had different goals, but everyone had the same need for health and well-being. The understanding and support we had for one another was tremendous.

Learning how to weight train properly and live a bodybuilder lifestyle has been incredible for me. It is all doable. The habits they've laid out, taking the steps—just keeping yourself on track. The science of changing your body with weight training and manipulating meals by adjusting macros to attain goals is captivating. There's a lot of measuring, but I find it interesting and fun. It's not always smooth going. It's more like a jerky progression of building blocks, learning curves with training, eating habits, sleeping habits, drinking water—until finally, you don't have to think about any of it.

It's all a learning process. It's about asking what's possible in each moment for all of us, taking a chance, showing curiosity. Anything is an opportunity to learn, grow, and help others and inspire them. For me, that instinctual reaction, that's big. Follow it and don't hold yourself back. Fall forward. When you start thinking you can't do it, catch yourself—they're just thoughts. Be optimistic and patient with yourself. How would you talk to a friend? Do that for yourself. Be encouraging to yourself because self-care is critical. Be your own great coach!

INDEX